Cutting Up

Laughing & Crafting

Ideas That Helped One Teenager Through Cancer Treatment

CREATED BY,

AUBRIE MAZE

FOR QUESTIONS, COMMENTS AND

FURTHER INFORMATION:

WWW.AUBRIESPAGE.COM

D0619228

First Created for Senior Project at Sonoma Valley High School: 2001 - 2002

First Handmade Editions: 2003

First 100 Handmade Books Sold!: January 2004

Ongoing Handmade Books Available Throughout the Year

Off to the Professionals!: October 2004

Cover picture:

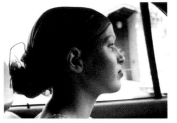

May 2001, driving home after having my "hair" and makeup
done for Junior Prom...in between chemo treatments!

ISBN 0-9763434-0-1

AMazing Publications

337 West Napa Street, Sonoma, CA 95476 USA

www.aubriespage.com

Copyright © 2004, Aubrie Maze and her licensors. All rights reserved. No part of this book may
be reproduced, stored in a retrieval system, or transmitted in any form or by any means without
written permission from the publisher.

Printed in China

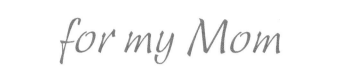

for my Mom

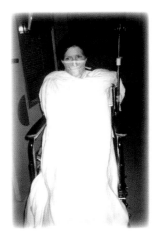

(Honestly)

It's okay to be pissed off.

I know I was.

It'll even do you good. It shows that you have the passion to live and the determination to fight. I know I wasn't always the most pleasant to be around, but that was during the times I had to turn inside myself to find that place where I could clench my teeth and battle my way through the poison (ie chemo) circulating in my body. I'm so grateful that those around me, mostly my parents, didn't take my irritability personally.

But I wasn't always so pissed off and such a pain to be around. That was only one aspect of my fight. It was also important to focus on anything and everything positive that would lift my spirits. So that's what this book is about—finding and focusing on the little things that make you smile, the little things that make each day go by a little smoother, that will lighten your heart, bring you joy, and eventually bring you to Remission.

While laughter cannot replace chemo, it's importance is definitely up there.

...just laugh.

How to Use This Book

In the following pages of this book, you will find a compilation of ideas gathered through the guidance of my parents, family, caretakers and friends. I hope these ideas that helped me so much in my journey through treatments will help you in your journey, or at least serve as a springboard for inspiration of your own ways to reach complete wellness.

You can use this book in any way you choose. Please, paste over my stuff, copy pages or cut it all up! This is YOUR book. Make it _yours_.

Most of all... Enjoy!

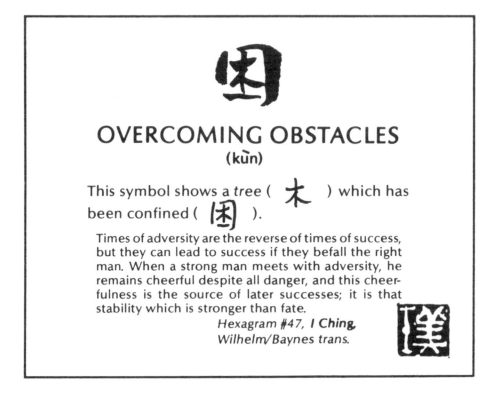

OVERCOMING OBSTACLES
(kùn)

This symbol shows a *tree* (　木　) which has been confined (　困　).

Times of adversity are the reverse of times of success, but they can lead to success if they befall the right man. When a strong man meets with adversity, he remains cheerful despite all danger, and this cheerfulness is the source of later successes; it is that stability which is stronger than fate.

Hexagram #47, I Ching, Wilhelm/Baynes trans.

A **CARAVAN** ® Storycard

my mom's story

Dear Fellow Travelers,

Here you stand, at the beginning of a journey on an unforged path. We know that you and your circumstances are unique, so we are only sharing our journey, offering some guidance and spirit of hope, knowing all too well, through our own experiences, that no one can really relate to what you are going through right now. Our hope is to help, if just a little. This is the toughest letter I've ever written and I am still nervous I didn't get it right. I will trust it is, so here we go.

Our daughter, probably much like your child, was a typical teen going through high school. It was May and she was looking forward to the end of her successful sophomore year. She had been studying hard, contributing to her high school Leadership Class, preparing for the driver's test, working her part-time job and hanging out with her friends. Soon to follow would be a fun filled summer: a family vacation, driving her very own wheels and practicing tennis with her high school team. She was having a blast.

And then **wham**, that little thing that had been bugging her on her left hip? The dull ache we were sure was just growing pains? That area below the iliac crest where a basketball happened to smack during a freezing 7 AM P.E. class? The ache no yoga stretch could affect, no osteopath, no shiatsu or massage practitioner could ease? That increasing pain the orthopedist called bursitis six weeks after her snowboarding fall, (where she landed right on it), but the physical therapist the next day suspected otherwise and joined me in nagging the orthopedist for two weeks for an MRI? That suddenly, strangely swelling hip? A TUMOR. It was a nightmare we would surely wake from...wouldn't we?

And then even worse news arrived. Further testing showed the cancer had metastasized to her lungs. I remember whispering a scream into the phone, "How can this be?"

With Aubrie passed out on Vicodin, I slowly came completely undone. I lost all strength to hold myself upright, even to breathe. I don't know how my husband, Aubrie's dad, Rick, held himself together, but thank God he could. I wanted to die. I couldn't do this. I felt a huge magnet sucking me to the couch. I stared at my girl lying there across from me. All my beliefs I had ever lived by evaporated leaving me with nothing to hold on to. Thank God for Rick's intervention and insistence. Through it he connected me with the perfect woman; his Mom, whose love for Aubrie was close to my own. We cried together for awhile and through her soothing voice and loving faith the grip of the magnet began to release me; through this release I was able to drop to my knees, praying for and gathering more strength.

In disbelief, we looked upwards towards our faith. This was not so easy right now. We asked ourselves and yelled at God, "Why her?" Noises went through my head like static from a radio station out of tune trying to hear the voice of guidance. We fought for understanding. I was so angry with myself for missing this. **How could I miss this?** My own guilt trying to consume me, I prayed – I screamed – for peace within myself, too.

You know, we all come to crossroads in our lives, that moment of choice where things are not so clear; this was one of ours. We had to choose our context and direction, and fast. Diving headfirst into the profound unknown we chose to trust Aubrie's new doctor and with her leadership we found our team of caretakers. In that profound unknown, like floating in a large ocean, we found our many angels, miracles and guides pointing the way. "Just put one foot in front of the other," they said and moment-by-moment, we found our ground. We found our deeper selves, too. The foundation to our faith grew stronger still, our faith in humankind and kindness was confirmed, and we found out how loved we were, not only by our family, but also by our friends and community. **We found that the degree to which one is challenged, to that degree is the blessing.**

I don't know why Aubrie got to heal so brilliantly, beating all those slim odds while others do not; only God knows. I had to reach deep and discovered the belief that whatever happened was between Aubrie and God; their deal together. I came to trust that which I cannot see and believe it is ultimately good. I did add a clause, a plea-ful request; If I had any vote the vote would be to have Aubrie as my daughter for a very, very long time.

We trusted the process to the best of our ability, became good team members, helped Aubrie and ourselves view life optimistically, looking for the gift of any given moment. We didn't know if we were having our last days with Aubrie or not, but we took no chances. Early on in her treatments she was depressed and grouchy, especially towards me. Sound familiar? Couldn't blame the kid, but I spoke to her quietly about how rare it was for any mother to get to spend this much time with her sixteen year old daughter and that I, for one, wanted to have fun doing it. She read between the lines, bolted upright in her hospital bed spitting words with pure certainty, "I'm NOT doing to **die**, Mom!"

Adopting **that** as our attitude, (whew!), we managed to bring fun, somehow, during or after any given episode. (Though, I'll admit, witnessing her vomit up baseball-sized blood clots was nowhere **in** my imagination at the time I made that original declaration...I didn't even know it was possible.) The nurses were great leaders at making gross things funny. They have had much more practice. We decided there is a special place in Heaven for those pediatric oncology nurses. I cannot imagine getting through those days without their spirit.

My husband and I leaned on each other. We took turns being each other's rock. We had different strengths. He could hear things I simply could not hear, I asked questions he simply could not ask. As we naturally sorted out our roles, he became **funny daddy**, I became **the general**. We stuck together, though it wasn't always easy. We knew Aubrie needed both of us to fight for her life. Somehow we found ways to have compassion for one another instead of taking our fears out on the other. We were both scared to death. We comforted each other.

Though I would have never chosen this painful path for my daughter, the young woman that emerged on the other side is a true warrior. She has developed a new strength and love, an intuition and focus formed through her journey that will serve her forever. She is a beacon of hope for others, a ray of sunshine that lights up the hearts of all who know her. I tease her it's all the radiation she received!

Oh, a few words on those "slim odds" and statistics you may be hearing about? As horrible and gut wrenching as they are, please remember one thing; your child is his or her own number. No matter what the scary voice is trying to tell you. Even in the slimmest of odds, which we came to embrace, someone comprised those small numbers, too. We grew to know and love slim odds. We **are** slim odds. Slim odds gave us something to "choose." The doctors would give us the scenario of the moment and, in our heads, we would make our selection. This became a regular game between Aubrie and me. (And was not something we shared out loud to many.)

Even if they tell you there are zero odds in your favor, know that we have witnessed children becoming the very first ever in areas of healing, creating new numbers for those stat lovers. Why not your child, too? We also grew accustomed to hearing, "Wow, never seen **that** before." For example, a rash from Emla cream, or her own unique right shoulder and arm deadening reactions to Benedryl, and my personal favorite, Decadron, which rendered her a temper-tantrum throwing two year old. And, 'that' also included when her lungs miraculously healed after whole lung radiation, without the usual steroids. It, too, gave us all something to marvel at. We may soon find pictures of her lungs with and without the B.O.O.P (and inflammation of the lung's lining) in a medical journal. The human body is a wonder.

We hope this book helps you. It has been healing to create. In these pages are keys to our daily codes, our routines, how we managed to keep an eye for the future, always dangling 'carrots' to move towards. I highly recommend 'dangling carrots.'

I wrote a poem, of sorts, for the times my inner-critic tried to get the best of me, tried to get me to rescind my role as the data collector, the fact finder, the one who sat through every AM and PM shift gathering evidence, seeing it all.
This is what I have to say to that –

Maybe I am the ultimate cheerleader
Maybe I do think too much
Maybe I do ask too many questions
And maybe I am a royal pain in the butt
But one thing I know for sure;
I am not a quitter.
We come from a long line of warriors
May the legacy continue.

A piece of wisdom I'd like to leave you with:
Never doubt yourself. Trust your instincts and let them guide you.
Never follow blindly. Ask respectful, thoughtful questions. You know your child.
And above all, keep good contact with God.

I was amazed; after all that screaming and yelling at God, when the static cleared He was still there. I guess He doesn't take things personally. Like my big sister tells me, He has really big shoulders.

May you be blessed on your journey.

Kristin Maze
Aubrie's Mom

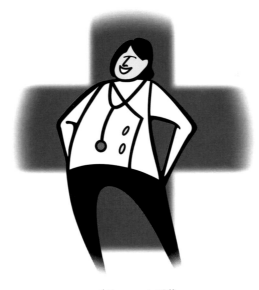

(Super MD!)

my doctor's story

I remember the first time I spoke with Aubrie on the telephone in May 2000. I had received a call earlier that day from the bone surgeon who specializes in tumors at UCSF about her case. He called to refer her for further treatment of a large Ewing's Sarcoma on her pelvis that had been giving her a lot of pain for several months. Despite the tremendous pain she was feeling from a cantaloupe-sized tumor on her left side, she was easy to speak with and understood everything I was telling her that needed to be done to complete her workup and start treatment. I could already tell on the phone that she was not a personality type to sit back and be passive—and she would later prove to be an active participant in her care with definite opinions and desires. Her parents were also the ideal advocates for her, always recognizing and respecting the conflicts between independence and dependence that challenge any adolescent, let alone one challenged with a life-threatening illness.

When I spoke with Aubrie on the phone that first evening, she had not yet had the baseline scan that would demonstrate areas of tumor spread in her lungs. I was honest with her, as I strongly believe that gentle honesty is the best way to forge a doctor-patient relationship, where my medical recommendations are always accompanied by some risk to my patient. I told her that we hoped that the tumor had not spread anywhere else but that our goal was to cure her of the disease, regardless of its location. So, when the results came back that the tumor had spread, Aubrie barely blinked and commenced the year-long journey to remission.

A cancer diagnosis is not just tragic because of the disease. It does not only invade someone's body but invades a person's daily life and that of their loved ones. In a very tangible way, it is incredibly inconvenient to have cancer. All of the other milestones and expectations, Thanksgiving at Grandma's, the Prom, Seth's graduation party, are secondary. Though there were many missed holidays and parties, Aubrie's family never lost sight of our goal—that staying on the course of therapy for the short term might help in the long term. They were also so lucky to have such a strong supportive network of family and friends that could help throughout the year. Lean on those people that can help—isolation adds unbearably to one's burden.

The year I spent with Aubrie and her family was like a trek I had made in the Himalayas—a half mile up, a quarter mile back, another half mile up, another quarter mile back. Every part of the journey needed to focus on something positive, something achieved, whether it was alleviating her pain early on or seeing her tumors melt away after the first two courses of chemotherapy. Little achievements add up to big ones, and if you can keep your mind positive, see the sunshine in your bleakest moments, and keep the overall goal always in sight, you, too, will be as well prepared as Aubrie to navigate the arduous road to recovery.

Doctor Mignon Loh, UCSF Children's Hospital Pediatric Oncologist

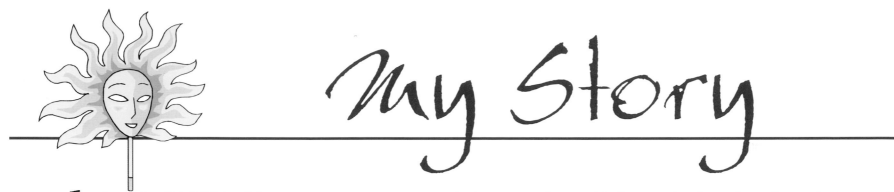

My Story

The date May 25, 2000 will forever stay in my memory as the beginning of a new life for me; the date of my diagnosis. It was the start of over a year's worth of cancer treatments, and the beginning of a new way of thinking, a new way of living.

In March of my Sophomore year of high school, I had a snowboarding accident on a Leadership class trip. My resulting swollen hip baffled everyone for eight weeks. As the swelling from the fall receded, it became apparent that something abnormal was growing on my hip. Between the persistence of my mom and my new physical therapist, an MRI appointment was arranged.

My parents and I were sent to Mount Zion Hospital in San Francisco after the MRI revealed a strange mass on my pelvis. We sat in disbelief and utter fear as the doctor started using the word "tumor." (Sheer confusion running through my head, "Wait...doesn't tumor have something to do with cancer?") Our worlds were turned upside down. Cancer suddenly felt so foreign and I realized I knew nothing about it. It was confirmed later that the mass on my pelvis was Ewing's Sarcoma, an aggressive form of bone cancer; it had also spread to my lungs, classifying me a "Stage Four."

My initial reaction to the doctor that day was pure quizzical curiosity. Before I could be afraid or even angry, I first needed INFORMATION...the facts. One of my first questions was if I was going to lose my hair. Losing my hair was the most tangible thing I could grasp, and it became my first reality and first opening for release of tears. As the hours passed on, I don't think I had any other feelings besides shock, fear and disbelief, as I sat crying; shaking and nauseous. The anger, depression, self pity, optimism and laughter would all come later. Each emotion played an important role in my recovery, each at the appropriate time.

Tears uncovered my first layer of acceptance. I made a conscious decision to do anything it took to beat my cancer. It was this initial reaction that was the pillar of my determination to live and my determination to have the best possible quality of life during my treatments.

At the start of my chemo, I was far from being all smiles, and I think it's perfectly normal and healthy to be angry at first. It shows the passion to live and the determination to fight. I know I wasn't always the most pleasant to be around, but that was during the times I had to turn inside myself to find that place where I could clench my teeth and battle my way through the poison circulating in my body. This anger was not constant; it was only one aspect of my fight. It was also important to focus on anything and everything positive that would lift my spirits.

For as long as I can remember, my relationship with my mom has been amazing (except for that one dark eighth grade year we don't talk about...); she is my mentor, advocate, best friend, and inspiration in every aspect of my life. Throughout all my treatments, whether I was in the hospital receiving chemotherapy or at home recuperating, my mom did something everyday to boost my spirits and keep them up. She knew exactly how to support me through my best and worst, and has a big enough heart to love me not only through the light-hearted, fun times, but also through the many occasions when I just needed to vent my anger and frustrations (towards her, of course.) My dad also played a large role in my optimism. He was my humor and could always make me laugh. He searched far and wide to come up with exciting foods and drinks to encourage my appetite, and he came up with goofy entertainment to keep me away from depression. Both of my parents were vital as constant advocates in the hospital and we reminded each other, if one of us forgot, to focus on anything and everything positive. They would very often ask me to tell them three things I was grateful for that day. This forced me to look at the bigger picture by being grateful for aspects of my life in degrees of relativity; maybe I was grateful that I wasn't feeling as sick as the day before, or that the pain caused by the expansion of my tumor was less. The more I practiced verbalizing my gratitudes, the more I realized how many aspects of my life there were to be grateful for.

The attitudes taken by my family, as well as their resulting support, were vital to my well-being. My older brother, Seth, was the first person to verbalize our optimism. After absorbing the shock of my diagnosis, he told me this was "just a bump in the road" and nothing to stop me from living; his practicality was refreshing. My grandmas, grandpas, aunts, uncles and cousins took turns flying or driving out to stay with our family. They took care of us and our home, making it possible for us to safely focus on our new responsibilities. My Grandma Maze, in particular, was a life saver. She practically moved in with us and, as my mom says, "held the mom space." She was, and still is, amazing. My extended family was just the beginning of those to help; our community rose to the occasion of helping out our family while in need. People wanted to help us; it made them feel useful and it lightened our burden. My girlfriends stayed at my side and supported me with all their hearts. Our bond is unbreakable.

My spirituality has shown me that everything is a gift from God as an opportunity to help us grow. I realized, at some point in my journey, with my parents' guidance, that I was responsible in allowing my bout with cancer to make me truly appreciate life. My experience with cancer was a gift as well as an obstacle, but never the less an experience that has tested and strengthened my mind, body and spirit.

I survived eleven months of chemotherapy, a major pelvic replacement surgery (as well as several "minor" surgeries), two weeks of whole lung radiation, and all the side effects of these treatments. The last step in the completion of my battle with cancer was on July 6, 2001 when I had a final surgery to remove my broviac, the central catheter I had lived with for over 13 months. I was declared in remission and moved from the world of cancer patients to the world of cancer survivors! I took an experience that I could have taken with bitterness and resentment and turned it into an opportunity to grow. I saw my community pause in their lives and give generously to my family. My family and I learned to speak up for what we needed in the hospital, and now in life. We believe in ourselves more. Our bond was strengthened to the degree only possible with such a trial. I learned the power of gratitude and perseverance with a positive outlook and plan to share my newfound knowledge with others.

...So that's what this book is about – finding and focusing on the little things that make you smile, the little things that make each day go by a little smoother, that will lighten your heart, bring you joy, and eventually bring you to Remission.

Enjoy...craft your own journey...and laugh lots.

Aubrie Maze

First of all...

I have found that writing my journey down on paper helped me tremendously. Not only did it help make my unreal situation feel more realistic, but it also is a great record to look back on when you're out of treatments, and a great set of milestones to mark how far you've come. After being on so many (legal) drugs, I forget much of what I went through. So when I read back on my thoughts, they seem almost foreign to me. Although I was scared and confused in some of my journal entries, it is (in a sick-humor sort of way) fun to be back inside that frame of mind, knowing now that everything turned out okay in the end. It is bizarre to know that subjects of which I wrote so intimately, I now have no recollection of except in my journal.

From my experiences, I would HIGHLY recommend that you keep a journal and take many pictures. I made this book so you could begin your own collection of pictures, writing, and various other bits of information. I especially enjoyed creating a scrapbook of cards, pictures, and various memorabilia. It was fun and creative, and even became a nice, new hobby. You may not always feel like being photographed, but it is important to keep a little silliness in your life, especially during cancer treatments. Remember that. In addition, the pictures are also really fun to look back on later when you forget the depth of your journey! During my treatments I felt sick, but only now, looking back, do I realize how truly sick I was. (I hate saying "sick" because I remember always being offended when people said I was "sick" or "ill." My reaction was always, "I don't have the flu...I'm not sick, I have cancer.") I was so brave.

...start with this simple writing and acceptance:

My name is

I am   years old

I was diagnosed with

on

The hospital I go to is

My Doctor's name is

My Diagnosis

The following was my first journal entry, telling the story of my diagnosis. I find it very interesting how detached I sound. I was in such shock, that I was just telling the story. I had no emotional attachment to the situation because its impact had not yet set in.

"...I want to keep a journal of everything that happens, for two reasons. First is that maybe someday this will help someone else going through what I'm going through now. Second, it's great for my sake—I can let out and release so much. It always makes me feel better when I write.

Towards the beginning of this year (January 2000) my left hip had been sore. We thought nothing of it—my dad was convinced it was growing pains... everyone said to just give it time.

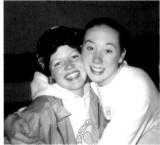

March 24-26 was the annual Leadership Ski trip to Squaw Valley. This was an event that every Leadership student looked forward to. We left Friday, shortly after school got out.

That night we got settled in our "Youth Hostel" and everyone hung out. Early the next morning we all set out to ski or snowboard. I chose to snowboard...long story short: we were killing time (us amateurs) before our lessons. I wiped out. And that snow was not soft. So I was carried away by ski patrol, and taken to the ER.

Lauren Flaherty stayed with me for the hours I was in the ER. I had my hip X-rayed, and all they said was it "looked" like nothing was broken, and I left with a pair of crutches. My entire left leg was in pain, but the worst seemed to be my hip—the same hip that had been bothering me since January. What are the odds of that? (Fate)

Seth [my older brother] happened to be there, too, though not with Leadership. That was very fortunate, and he took me home that night. I missed two more days of so much fun: more skiing/snowboarding, sledding, ice-skating, swimming, and late night "parties!"

(3/27) A day or so after I was home, my mom took me to see an Osteopath recommended to us by several people. I went in sobbing my little heart out—it hurt even to stand. I was under his care for about an hour. He was so amazing—a miracle worker. I walked out of that place in almost no pain, just a strong limp.

I spent a full week out of school—on Vicodin. So I basically slept for a week.

The month of April was pretty much dedicated to my hip problem. No one knew what was really going on, but I stayed gimpy and pretty anti-social. I went to a few Shiatsu treatments, and that was great. We decided it was probably my sciatic nerve—the main nerve of the leg. My hip was greatly "swollen" and we decided that my muscle was in spasm.

On May 4—from major persuasion from my mom, my daddy took me to see the osteopath. He was amazed I wasn't better after more than a month. Healthy, young people are usually cured within two visits—I wasn't. He also said if it was Sciatica, he didn't want to mess with it—obviously not his area of expertise. So he sent us to an Orthopedic Surgeon in Sonoma. Luckily, we were able to get in that same day, around 4:00 pm.

I put on a gown, and he made a quick decision. Too quick in my opinion. He pushed on my leg, and moved it around a bit. From that little bit of information, he "knew" it was bursitis. I didn't trust the way he so quickly shot down any other possibilities. Later I realized I should have trusted my instincts.

The doctor sent me to Physical Therapy for two weeks, after which I would come back to see him. I'm not sure the few times I went did much. But Justin (my Physical Therapist) was the one who insisted something wasn't right. He and his co-workers were confused by my combination of symptoms.

When I went back to the Orthopedic Surgeon on Thursday, May 18th, I pointed out my swollen hip. He was very concerned and scheduled me for an MRI the next Wednesday (May 23rd). That wasn't so scary—since I'm claustrophobic, and, therefore, was able to be in an "open" MRI machine. The doctors there couldn't tell us anything, but we had an appointment with the Orthopedic Surgeon that afternoon .

The Orthopedic surgeon looked over my MRI's, talked to us (just me and mom), and then we saw it. There was a huge grapefruit sized mass in my pelvic area. [Measuring 22cm in one direction.] He said it could be many things, probably harmless, though worst possible scenario it could be a tumor. We took that out of our minds since we thought it was a highly unlikely chance.

By another miracle, we were able to get an appointment with Dr. James Johnston, an Orthopedic Oncologist (bone cancer specialist) the very next day.

Thursday the 25th of May, we drove to the city, to Mount Zion. We waited about two hours, and I got really frustrated.

Oops—I forgot to say that Dr. Johnston is literally the best doctor in the world—in his specialty! There are four doctors (orthopedic oncologists) in the US that are the best in the world. One lives in NY, one in Florida, one in Texas, and one here in SF!

So I was tired of waiting, maybe not ready to go through what I was about to go through. When he finally came in, he started talking. During his talking he made a casual reference to "my tumor"—maybe assuming we already knew. We didn't even put it together (at least I didn't) that his specialty was bone cancer. That was traumatizing. I was shocked—it so didn't feel real.

He talked to us more in detail about my cancer, and we asked a lot of questions. Before he could be positive about this whole thing, the next step was to walk a block to visit another doctor. He did some tests on me. He shot me right in my tumor mass with some numbing stuff, then stuck a huge needle in and took out some cells of my tumor. I can comfortably say "my tumor" now, a big step for me. For a while those two words hit me hard and made me cry.

So he took some more (two more) samples out of me, and filled the hole with some black powder so they would know where the needle had been. It's a permanent tattoo, but if I have surgery, they'll take out that little piece of skin.

The tests confirmed my exact type of tumor: Ewing's Sarcoma. It is most common in people under 30 years, and also most common in the hip area. It seems that mine is growing off my Iliac Crest (the bone that jabs out of your hip especially when you lay down...)

Then we went back to see Dr. Johnston again, just to clarify everything.

The next day—Friday the 26th I was scheduled for a couple tests at the Sonoma Valley Hospital. I had a bone scan, and a CT of my lungs. Even after the films were printed out, the hospital people couldn't tell us anything.

Dr. Mignon Loh—my main doctor, is amazing. She called me the first time on the 25th. I talked to her for 30 minutes the first time. She was terrific, and amazed at the questions I had to ask. ("How do you know to ask all of this?") She made sure I knew she was my doctor, not my parents'—and I could call her anytime and tell her anything.

So—after my CT and bone scan, she talked to the SVH doctors, and asked what they saw (she told them what to look for...). Then she called us. It didn't look like there were any tumor cells in my bone marrow—which would be the worst place. Bad news: the lung scan (CT) showed I did have spreading of my tumor to my lungs—but only in little pieces.

She told us that Saturday evening—the 27th."

I was scheduled to go in for broviac placement and chemo in a few days, but pain forced us in sooner: Memorial Day, May 29, 2000. My friends came to see me off, and then I spoke to Paul Crowe, a survivor of Osteo-Sarcoma. We made the drive to UCSF Medical Hospital where I was shot with morphine to ease my pain. The rest is blurry... but that day I started my first round (of many) of chemotherapy.

(write the story of your diagnosis here)

The Story of My Diagnosis:

Completely Hairless:

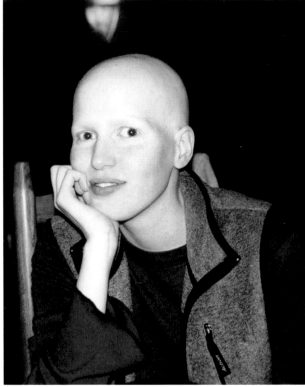

November 2000

A Full Head of Hair:

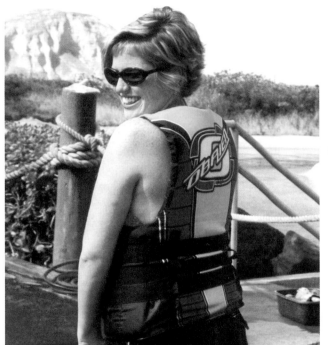

August 2003

(my Make-A-Wish trip to Hawaii!)

Being bald had its perks: I didn't have to worry about greasy hair when I couldn't get out of bed...it was a hassle to shower with my broviac, so shallow baths were ultimate...

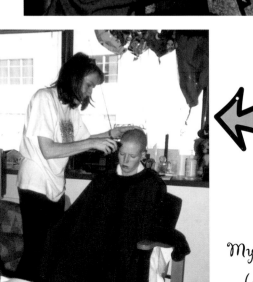

Round Two of Chemo...my mom shaving my head. Deciding to shave your head is an extremely difficult decision, but I think getting rid of it all at once is much easier than waiting out the gradual hair-loss process.

My mom doing my hair for Prom 2002 (almost one year after Remission!)

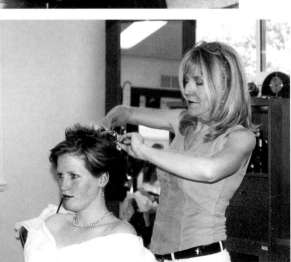

This is me with hair... 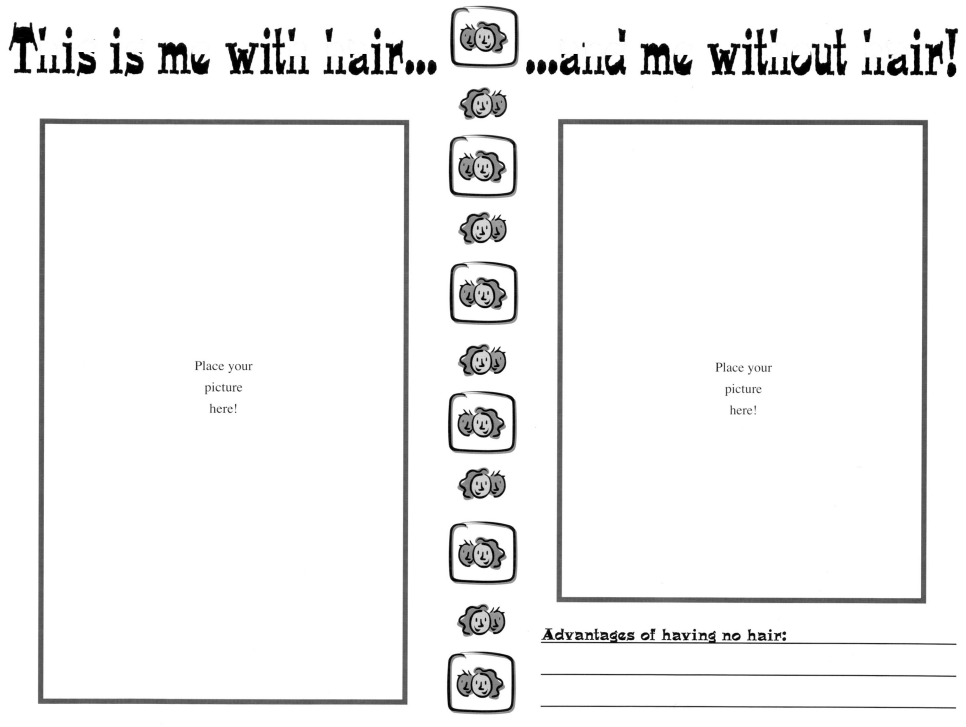 ...and me without hair!

Place your
picture
here!

Place your
picture
here!

Advantages of having no hair:

...CHOICE...

It is important to stay in choice.

To stay in choice is to choose the best for yourself and hold the vision that it will happen. When given two or more possibilities, hold the vision that the favorable one WILL prevail. Your mind will want to dwell on ideas, but why give credibility to a scary and hopefully not true one? Give your energy only to the one you want to see happen. Give it power and choose that it will happen. Affirmations are a huge part of choice. One fact that has stayed with me is about affirmations: it has been proven that repeated statements, whether good or bad, actually leave grooves in the brain. The "mind over matter" phrase is true! If you constantly focus on how sick you are, this is only aiding your cancer. If you tell yourself you are healthy, your body will believe it. You may be physically weak, but you will have an element to neutralize this: hope.

Trust your Doctors and remember that you are a team.
You are the major player in this fight for your life. Fight.
You are unique. Trust your instincts. Trust yourself.
Be one of the people who makes up the percentage of survivors.
Be the person to whom the Doctors and Nurses say, "Wow. I've never see _that_ before..."
Be what you want. Be your own statistic.
Hope. Dream. Survive.
Choose to stay in choice.

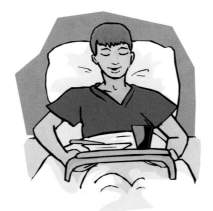

i am...

i choose...

Visualizations

I found that picturing visualizations (imagining your insides doing what you want) were extremely useful in my complete recovery. Most of my visualizations were created by Laura Dee, my "personal Shiatsu Master." My visualizations ranged in variety and purpose: from my butterfly visualization for my radiation (described below) to the simple movement of energy... When I was afraid to have my hip touched, fearing my replacement would fall apart, it helped to picture glowing balls of energy traveling up and down, across and though my hip to keep everything moving smoothly.

Before my tumor was surgically removed from my body, I pictured little "pacmen" circling through my hip eating and destroying any and all cancer cells. I drew a picture of this, shown on my "War Wounds" page.

Visualization ties right in with staying in choice, giving energy only to the good, not the bad. Dwelling on the negative only gives it power. Likewise, dwelling on the positive, having affirmations, gives power to the good. Even to visualize yourself out of treatments: decide to go somewhere and start planning the trip. It gives your mind something fun to dwell on, as well as tells your brain you WILL get better. Your subconscious has a hard time determining reality from imagination. Picture yourself at your ideal place in life (physically or emotionally)... and believe it.

An email written to friends and family:

May 3rd, 2001

Hi everyone! Well, today was my very last radiation treatment! I'm so excited. The radiation was fairly simple and harmless - it was the side effects that were tough. I had a rough time sleeping because I was up all night coughing - (the radiation directly hit part of my esophagus, making it raw and irritated). So that wasn't much fun. But my visualization was wonderful. Each morning I would allow beautiful rose petaled butterflies to float into my lungs. With their wings, they would sweep out anything unwanted. And the radiation was just sunlight to feed the butterflies. Anything bad coming from the radiation was also absorbed by the butterflies, not my lungs. Then the butterflies would put the icky part of the radiation into these little pouches. At the end of the day, I would release the butterflies, taking with them their little pouches. The next morning a new, fresh group of butterflies would be brought in to do the same job...and so on. The visualization was mostly thanks to the wonderful Laura Dee (thank you so much!).

Tuesday the 8th, I am scheduled to go in for my second to last chemotherapy treatment. Then the 10th is my 17th birthday!! How exciting. And my Grammie is coming from Wisconsin on my birthday. Oh, and then Prom is the 12th!!! I'll be having quite a busy couple of days...

SO - my hair is growing back!!! I'm not sure if it'll stay through these last two treatments, so I'm not getting too attached. But it sure is a fun, new feeling. I've got peach fuzz on my head, and even eyelashes and eyebrows! It's all such blonde, baby hair. And getting goosebumps with hair is such a foreign feeling - it actually brings me pain! Well, I'll sign off for now - I'll try to write again soon!

Thank you all for your great notes. Much love, Aubrie

.i visualize my body in total and perfect health.

Comparing Catheters

Aubrie Maze, age 19. Diagnosed with Ewing's Sarcoma at age 16. In remission! (Pictured both left and right.)

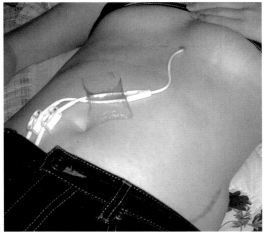
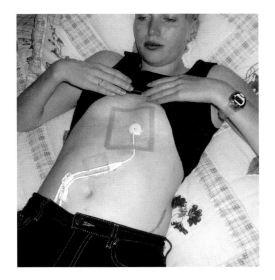

I had a broviac, and from my experience, I kind of enjoyed it. I rarely had to be injected with needles (which is just an added hassle!) I enjoyed being able to do my own blood draws; flushing and heparin-locking the line each night was fun most of the time (although I DO have a selective memory...) I felt like such a big kid! The most vulnerable I ever felt was each week when my mom would change the dressing on my site, and my worst fear became the thought of my line being ripped from my body...

I found that everything went hand-in-hand: I couldn't shower (without changing my dressing afterwards), but since I had no hair on my head, my daily shallow baths were sufficient, even perfect.

Justin Ono, age 18. Diagnosed with A.L.L. at ages 10, 13, and 16. Currently in treatments.

Justin says the pros of his port-o-cath are that he can swim and be active, and only has to flush his port once a month. The cons of his port are his "reduced physical abilities," meaning that his port "impedes [his] ability to truly sacrifice [his] body," thus preventing him from playing football. Justin is still able to wrestle and everyone knows to watch out for the metal disk in his chest. Obviously, Justin's energy has remained remarkably high through his chemo treatments!

Brent Zweigle, age 19. Diagnosed with Ewing's Sarcoma at age 19. Currently still in treatments.

"When I had a Hickman, it took a lot of time and patience to keep the Hickman comfortable and where it wouldn't bug me while it was not in use. It took time out of my day to keep it clean and not let it get an infection. I had to swab it with iodine three times, then put a patch over it and tape the sides down. That didn't work so well because the tape would lose it's strength and would just hang and be annoying.

"A month and a half before I got a port-a-cath, I started to use an Ace wrap and just wrap it around my body. It helped out a lot because it allowed my skin to heal from the tape I was using earlier to keep the lines up to my chest. The wrap was more comfortable because I didn't have to use tape or anything else.

"Having a port is a lot more comfortable, you only have to clean it when you take a shower (and you just shower regular, you don't even know it's there.) I had to flush the Hickman everyday (so the lines wouldn't get plugged up.) The port only has to be flushed once a month."

Megan Cates, age 20. Diagnosed with Yok Sac Tumors at age 17. In Remission!

"In my opinion broviacs are far more convenient than getting an IV every few days. I felt that having a broviac over IVs was that I could keep it in throughout my whole treatment. IVs can burst your vein and have to be redone and with broviacs that can't happen. I was terrified of the thought of needles, so when I heard the concept of a broviac I knew that it was for me. You can get all your treatments through a broviac: hydration, blood, chemo, and best of all PAINKILLERS! (haha) Some of the cons to a broviac is that it requires a surgery, it is painful for a little bit, sometimes it can take a little manipulation to get blood from it, and my mom says that the cleaning of it wasn't very fun either."

Jenny Ullman, age 20. Diagnosed with aplastic anemia at age 18. In Remission!

"When you have a blood disorder, the most important thing is getting access to the blood stream to provide treatment and to draw blood for constant revisal of your levels. In my case, the day that I arrived at the hospital for my treatment, they put in a catheter (thin plastic tube) that connected to the aorta. In the operation, they made a cut at the neck and installed a tube that strung down into the main artery right above the heart. They had to create an apparatus to keep the tube in place by securing it with four stitches into my neck area and sealing it from contact with water by putting on a transparent plastic bandage. The tube had three portals (place to connect it to a syringe or IV tube.) The point of having more than one was so that we would connect one portal to the IV tube where the medicines were coming in and at the same time the nurse could connect another portal to a syringe in order to take blood tests.

"The whole process of putting in the catheter took about an hour in an operating room downstairs and then I was back up in my room. My neck was sore for a while, I felt stiff, like if I moved even an inch the whole tube would come out, and my blood would go squirting everywhere. By the next day, I felt much better and I was so grateful for having it because they were not taking blood from the veins in my arm and wrists anymore. My arms really hurt after a month of diagnosis testing. My treatment only lasted a week in the hospital and then a few months of rest at home. I had the catheter in that whole time. At home, they taught us how to clean it by changing the bandaging every few days. I learned how to operate the portals myself which was an important part of the daily cleaning. Someone had to help me change the bandage. When they finally took it out a few months later, I felt as if I was missing something, but at least now, I have a scar to help me remember it."

My Catheter:

Taking Care of Myself

While it is important to trust your doctors and nurses, and let them take care of you, it is also important to watch out for yourself. You will find yourself in situations where you and your parents are the most experienced with how to take care of you, and often the most knowledgeable about your cancer. This can be in a local hospital, a hospital ward not specialized in oncology, and especially in your home. My parents were great in making sure my broviac was not mistreated in times when nurses and doctors were unexperienced with its correct usage, but I found there were times when I was without my parents and had to stand up for myself: I occasionally had to take over a blood draw or fluid flush in order to keep myself and my broviac safe. You are the only person always there to take care of yourself, so learn how to!

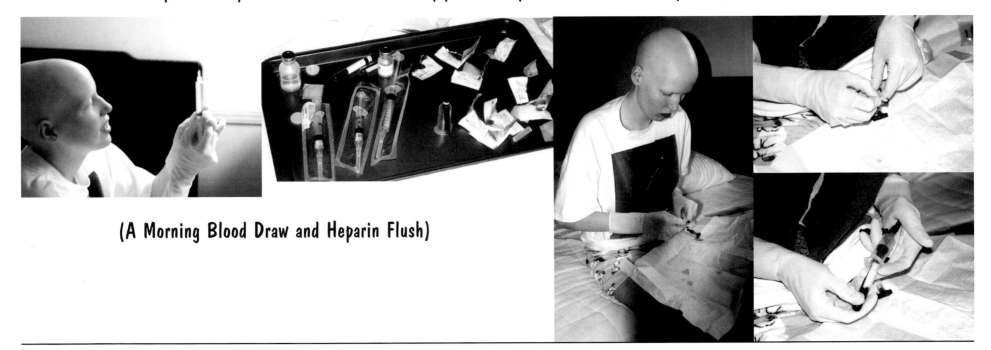

(A Morning Blood Draw and Heparin Flush)

for more on the science of these products, consult: www.glycoscience.com

Two dietary supplements I took regularly were glyconutrients and phytonutrients. The glyconutrients come in a powder form that contains all eight essential sugars, naturally occuring in nature, to aid in optimal cellular communication. My mom would sprinkle these glyconutrients, a tasteless powder, on everything I ate. I would also munch on phytonutrients (in the form of gummy bears), which contain dried fruits and vegetables. I loved their taste and they gave me the nutrients I was missing without sufficient food consumption. I truly believe that these products contributed greatly to my complete recovery.

How I Take Care of Myself:

positive affirmations

The poster on the next page was always up in the hospital rooms at UCSF Children's Hospital. I could look at this poster and see which face I most related to. This gave everyone around me an idea of how good or not-so-good I was doing, without actually having to describe myself.

I also found it beneficial to give myself positive affirmations. When anyone asked how I was feeling, my response would convey that I felt slightly better than I really did. If I was super bad, I would say I was "not so good." This way I never told myself I was doing bad. I kept telling myself I was a little better than I really was. And I believed myself. I usually said I was "okay." Once I really felt okay, I said I was "fine." Soon I was saying I was "good," and then "great." Now that I really am great, I say I'm "awesome" with a big smile!

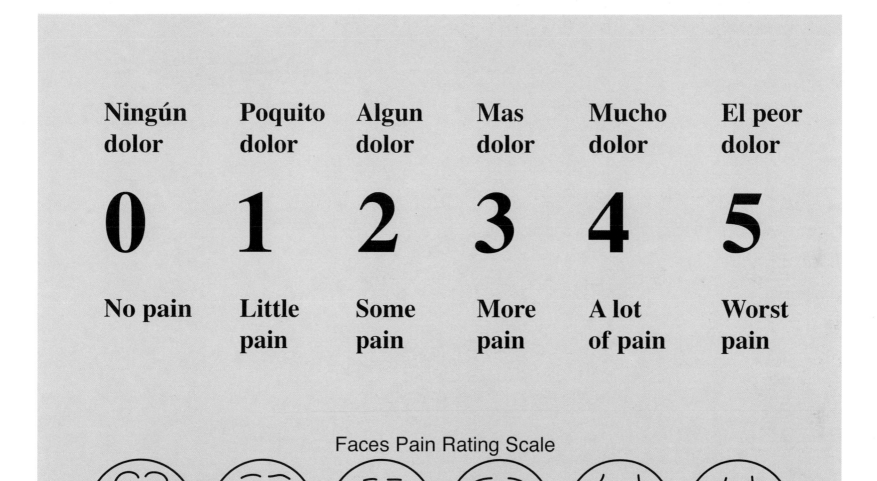

Ningún dolor	Poquito dolor	Algun dolor	Mas dolor	Mucho dolor	El peor dolor
0	**1**	**2**	**3**	**4**	**5**
No pain	Little pain	Some pain	More pain	A lot of pain	Worst pain

Faces Pain Rating Scale

Since you may be spending a lot of time in the hospital, it pays to make your hospital room feel like home. Bring pictures and favorite items from your room or house to fancy up your hospital room. (We always kept a second piece of luggage packed full of my little knick-knacks for the hospital.) Put a sign on your hospital room door that makes the room your own.

My big thing is to make the best of everything. Since I believed in living "day by day, moment by moment," it was important to make the best of those days and moments, even in the hospital.

(your hospital room)

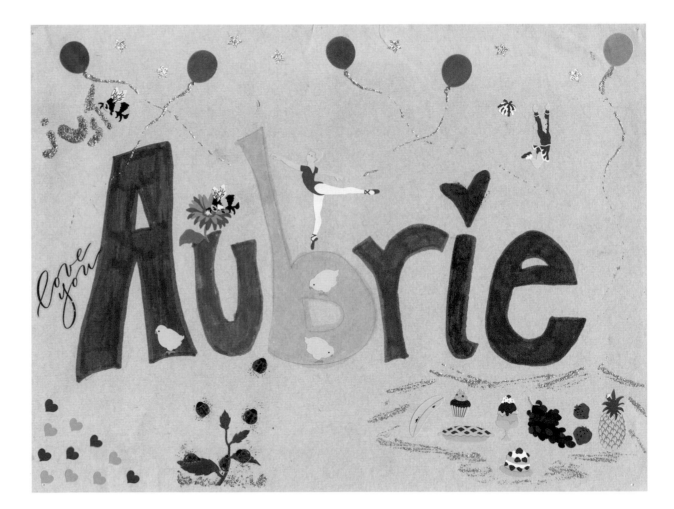

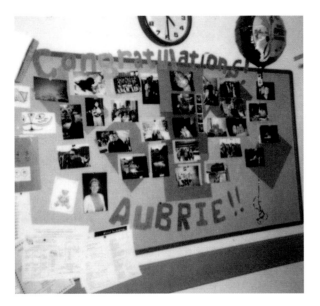

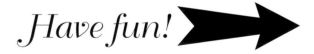

Have fun!

'S ROOM

Write down a list or compilation of things that bring you joy.

Use this list as a reminder of what will put a smile on your face for when you are feeling down.

What Makes Me Happy:

day:
Sunday
date:
6-18-00
time:
1:50

It's Father's Day! I'm at home and I'm feeling good (relatively).

What makes me happy:

Corey Haim's one-sided grin

Watch a funny movie when you're feeling down - it takes my mind off everything... my pain.

My Favorite Story:
A friend of ours, Laura Dee, raffled off her BMW, and the profits went to "Aubrie's Fund." Many of the people put my name on their ticket, so when my brother pulled the raffle ticket at a benefit variety show for me, it had my name on it! I won a beautiful red, convertible BMW!!!

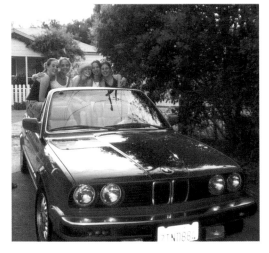

My Dad's Silliness:

Once my dad walked into my hospital room with a bag full of snacks (to get me to eat), with those wax Dracula teeth in his mouth. He walked around, talking to nurses, like everything was totally normal. He took everyone by surprise, even scared a few nurses! Everyone got a kick out of it. He brought humor to me and my mom as well as everyone on the hospital ward.

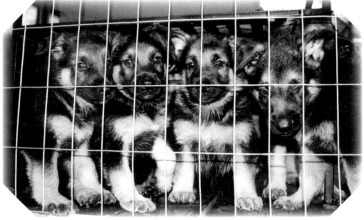

My Dog's Litter of Puppies – Summer of 2000

Music in my room

Drawing

Playing Wheel of Fortune on Nintendo

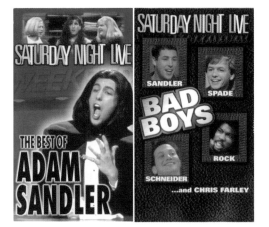

Adam Sandler & Saturday Night Live Reruns!!!

Things That Bring Me Joy

Some Senses

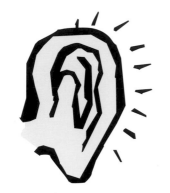

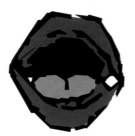

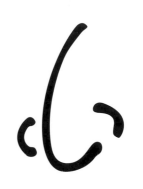

Among the huge suitcase of _stuff_ we always brought to the hospital was a boombox. Since the hospital never sleeps, we would sometimes play music around the clock. I loved listening to my favorite music while I was awake, and gentle music while I was sleeping. Music would cover the constant sounds of the hospital that might irritate me. And nurses loved hanging out in our room with the calm and interesting environment we created!

Just some things about food I want you to know:

It may become very difficult to eat, so anytime you feel you can eat, please do. And don't feel like eating is a wasted job if you throw up: some nutrients will absorb into your body. So keep eating – you need food and its nutrients to stay healthy!

Most any food you eat while in the hospital or anytime you are sick from treatments will attract a bad connotation. If you get sick from treatments and throw up a certain food, you may not want to eat that food again for a long time. Even though it is not the food that makes you sick, you may connect that food with being sick and/or vomiting. At first I didn't eat my favorite foods because I didn't want to develop bad connotations with them, but then it became important to eat <u>anything</u> I could.

Hospital smells can get disgusting especially with the lingering smells of vomit and bathroom voids (to be perfectly honest with you). When on chemo, I became extra-sensitive to any smell. Some reoccurring smells grossed me out, even when they were not gross smells. Along with the necessities we brought to the hospital, we would bring essential oils and good-smelling sprays. These helped so much even though I developed bad connotations with some of the smells. A good smelling room also attracted nurses to hang out with us!

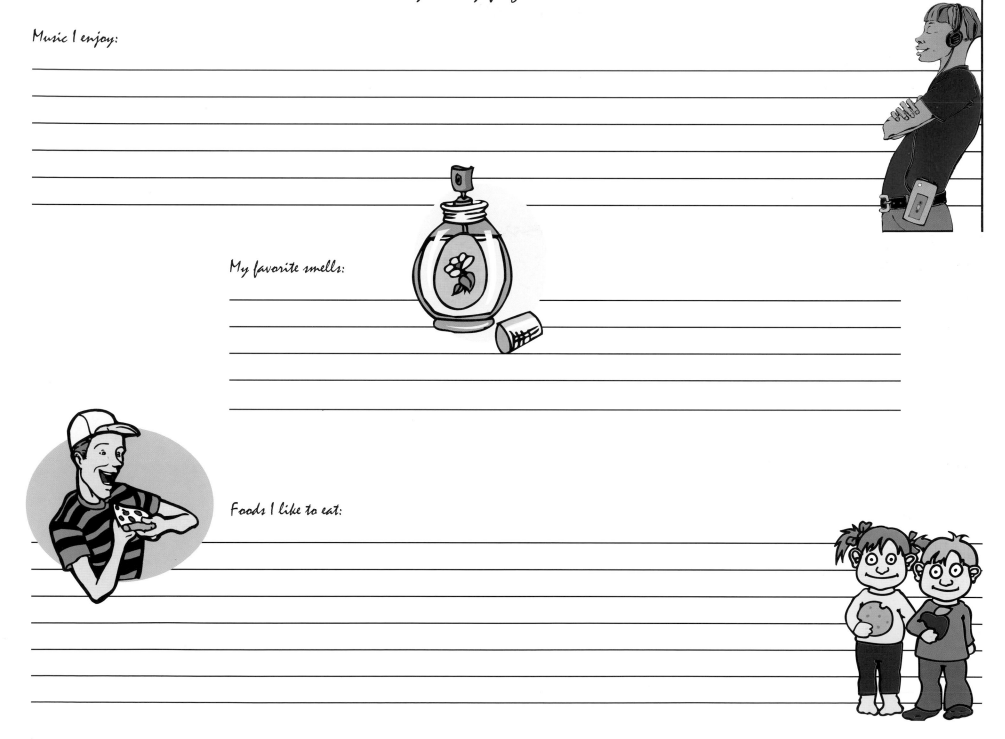

write these down because, trust me, you may forget!

Music I enjoy:

My favorite smells:

Foods I like to eat:

GRATITUDE

My parents made sure I found three things each day to be grateful for. I was irritated at their persistence, but it did help me put things on the "Relative Scale." I find it amazing that I found so much to be grateful for in a time of such tremendous...stuff. I always tried to not repeat things I had previously been grateful for, and I always picked my three best ideas, (as if I was limited to three!) There is so much in life to appreciate because any situation could always be worse. It is important to focus on what you have, not what you wish was different.

So on these following two pages, write each day three things you are grateful for. An example of my gratitudes are below.

> "Dear God –
>
> I am thankful for so much. I love you – Thank you for the sun.
>
> I am thankful that my foot hurts less (though still hurts!)
>
> I am thankful my throat hurts less.
>
> I am thankful my cancer is out of my lungs.
>
> I am thankful that my tumor is ever-shrinking.
>
> I am thankful for my amazingly supportive family!
>
> I am thankful I am not in need of a nose tube (though thankful for it probably saving my life)
>
> I am thankful to have the strength to live each day at a time."

Three things I am grateful for today:

1)_____

2)_____

3)_____

Three things I am grateful for today:

1)_____

2)_____

3)_____

Three things I am grateful for today:

1)_____

2)_____

3)_____

Three things I am grateful for today:

1)_____

2)_____

3)_____

Three things I am grateful for today:

1)_____

2)_____

3)_____

Three things I am grateful for today:

1)_____

2)_____

3)_____

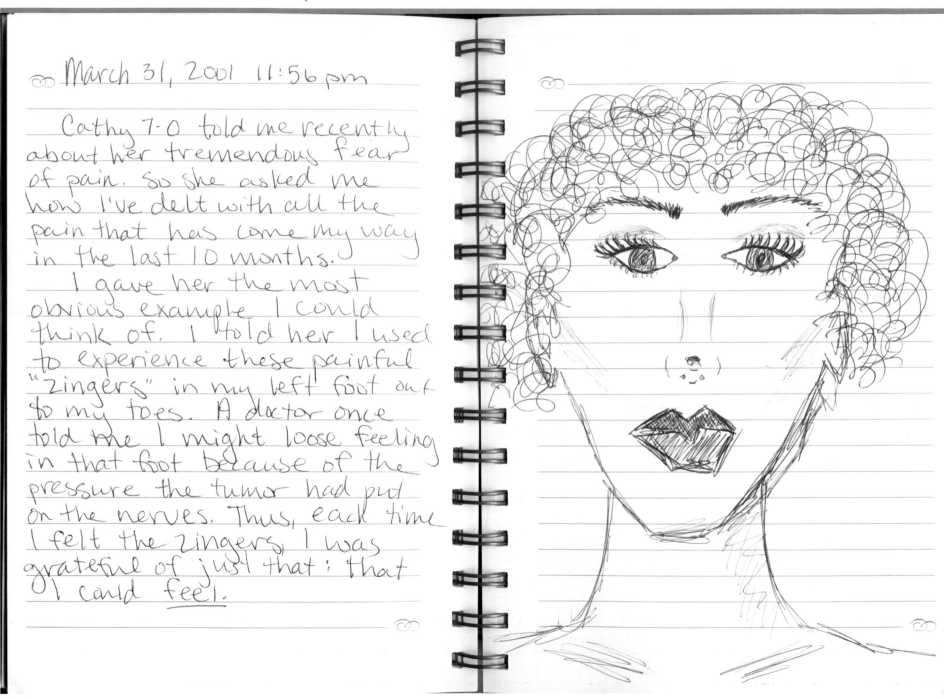

March 31, 2001 11:56 pm

Cathy 7-0 told me recently about her tremendous fear of pain. So she asked me how I've delt with all the pain that has come my way in the last 10 months.

I gave her the most obvious example I could think of. I told her I used to experience these painful "zingers" in my left foot out to my toes. A doctor once told me I might loose feeling in that foot because of the pressure the tumor had put on the nerves. Thus, each time I felt the zingers, I was grateful of just that: that I could feel.

Three things I am grateful for today:

1) _____

2) _____

3) _____

Three things I am grateful for today:

1) _____

2) _____

3) _____

Three things I am grateful for today:

1) _____

2) _____

3) _____

Three things I am grateful for today:

1) _____

2) _____

3) _____

Three things I am grateful for today:

1) _____

2) _____

3) _____

Three things I am grateful for today:

1) _____

2) _____

3) _____

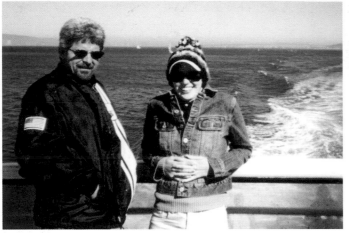

With my Dad in June 2001

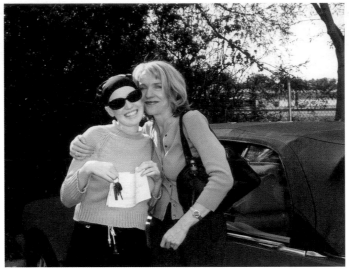

My Mom with me when I received my
official driver's liscense! October 2000

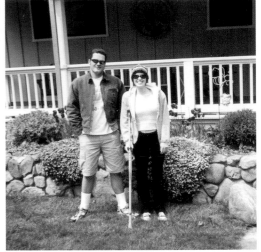

My brother and I visiting my
Grandparents, Spring 2001

MY FAMILY

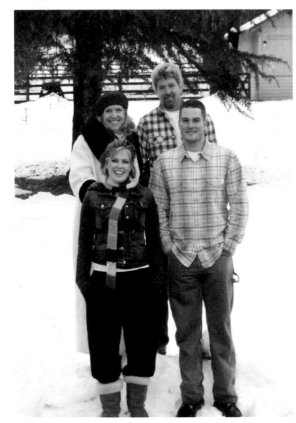

The four of us, Christmas 2003,
at my Grandparents' house

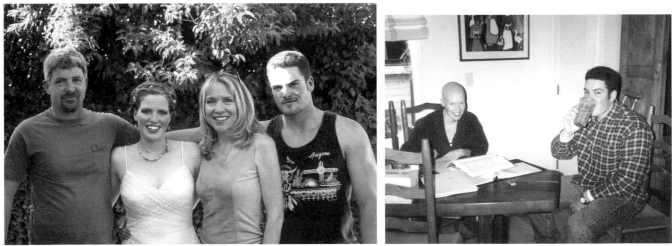

The four of us, May 2002, on my Prom Day

Getting Geometry help from my
older brother, Seth, in February 2001

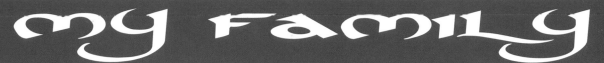

MY FAMILY

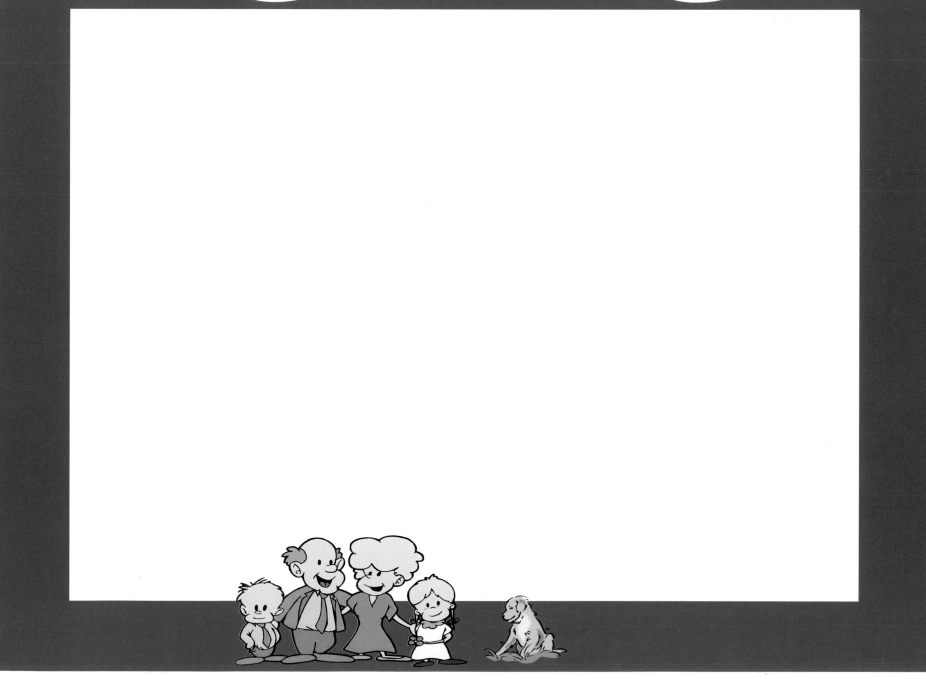

MY BEST FRIENDS...

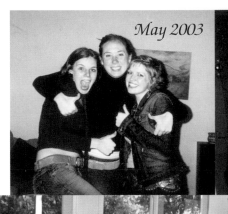
May 2003

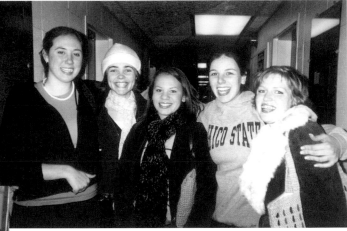
Visiting Chico State – February 2003

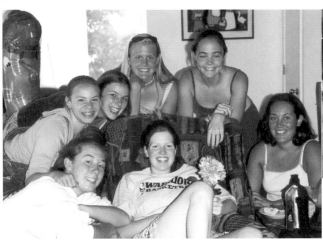

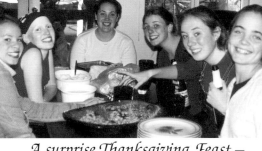
*A surprise Thanksgiving Feast –
November 18, 2000*

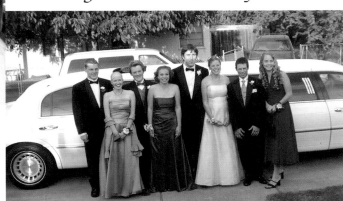
Junior Prom 2001 – in between chemo

*Just before I left for the Hospital the
very first time – May 30, 2000*

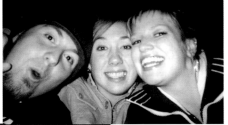
November 2003

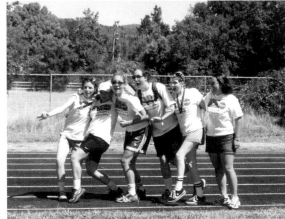
Relay for Life – August 2001

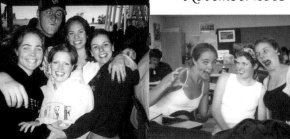

Spring Break 2002   *In Leadership 2001*   *At the beach – April 2002*

MY FRIENDS!

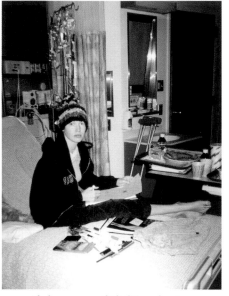

February 2001 – being crafty in the hospital

Me!

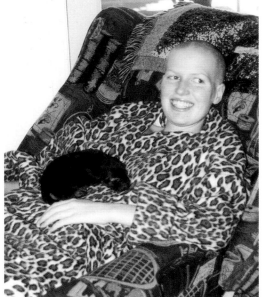

June 2000 – with one of my puppy's puppies!

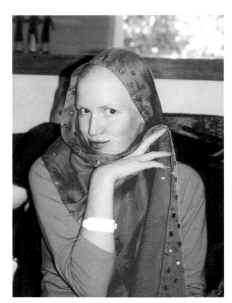

July 2000 – modeling a new scarf

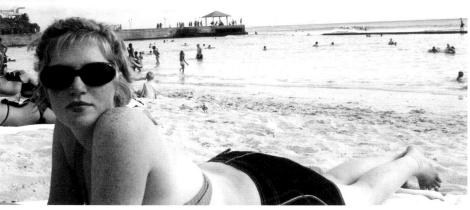

August 2003 – attempting a tan on Waikiki... with SPF 45, of course.

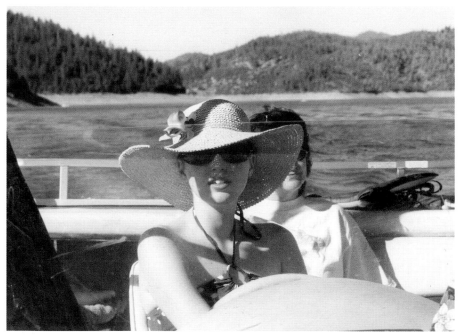

August 2001 – on the Trinity Lake

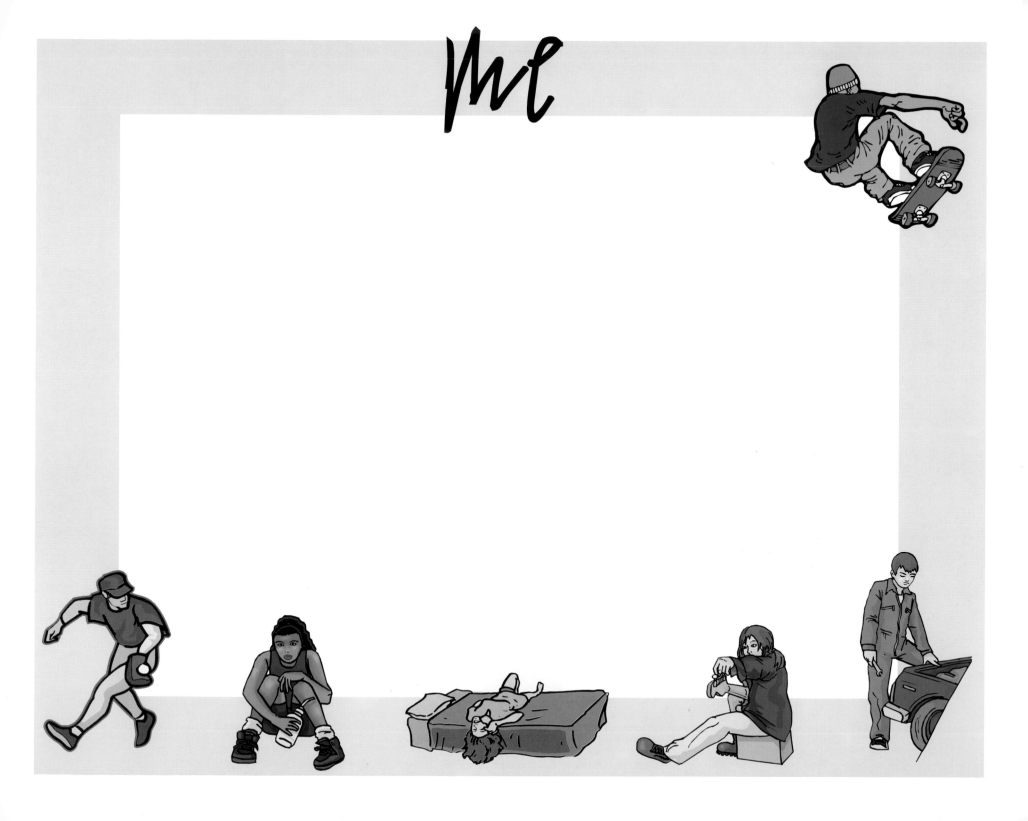

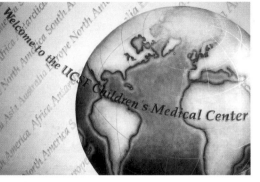

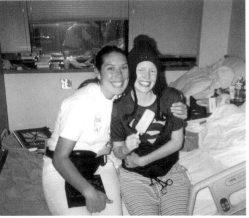

Erin Galvin, Registered Nurse

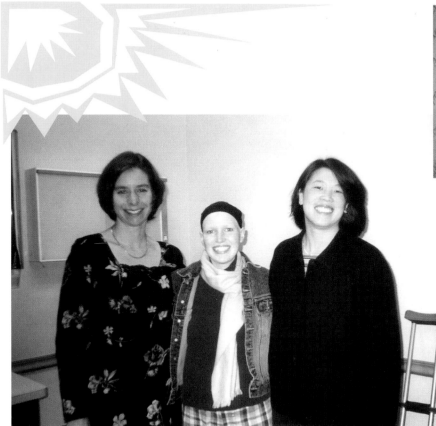

Dr. Daphne Haas Kogan,
Radiation Oncologist

Dr. Mignon Loh,
Pediatric Oncologist

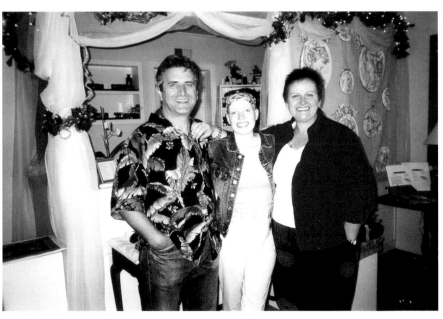

Gary Ruiz and Laura Dee Ruiz, Shiatsu Masters

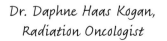

Three of my caretakers, including my
first nurse, Jim O'Brien and social worker
Beatie Lazard (right)

Some of
My Healers

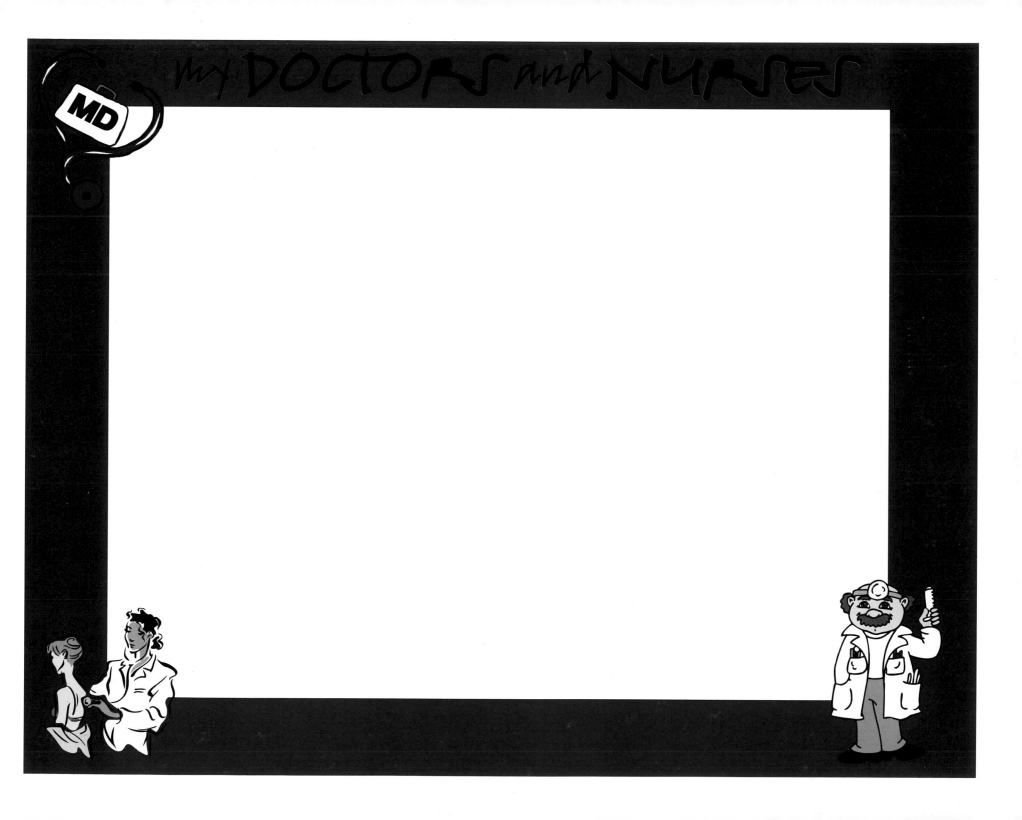

my DOCTORS and NURSES

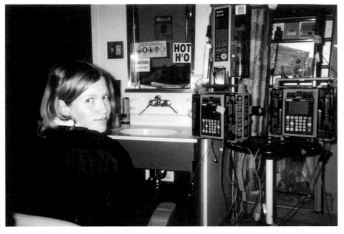

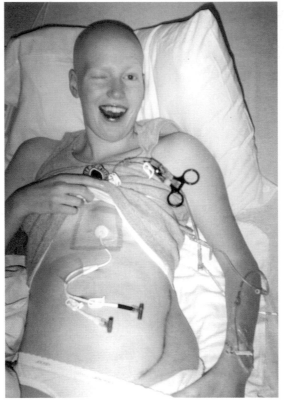

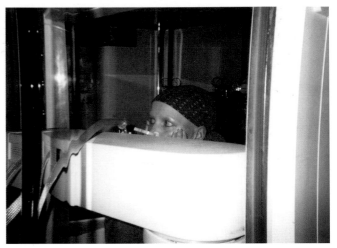

Scars are beautiful. They tell a story of you and your journey. Looking back on these pictures, it's hard for me to believe this was really me. I am proud of how I've gone through this battle, and I wear my scars with pride!

BATTLING CANCER:
MY WAR WOUNDS

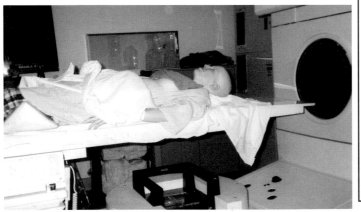

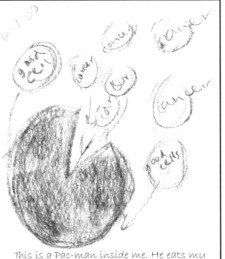

This is a Pac-man inside me. He eats my cancer cells and takes them to the center of the earth where they can be healed!

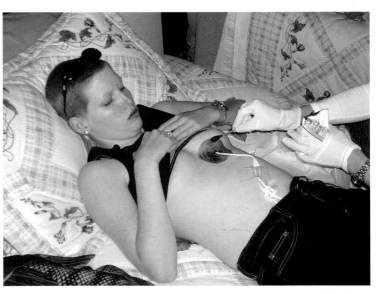

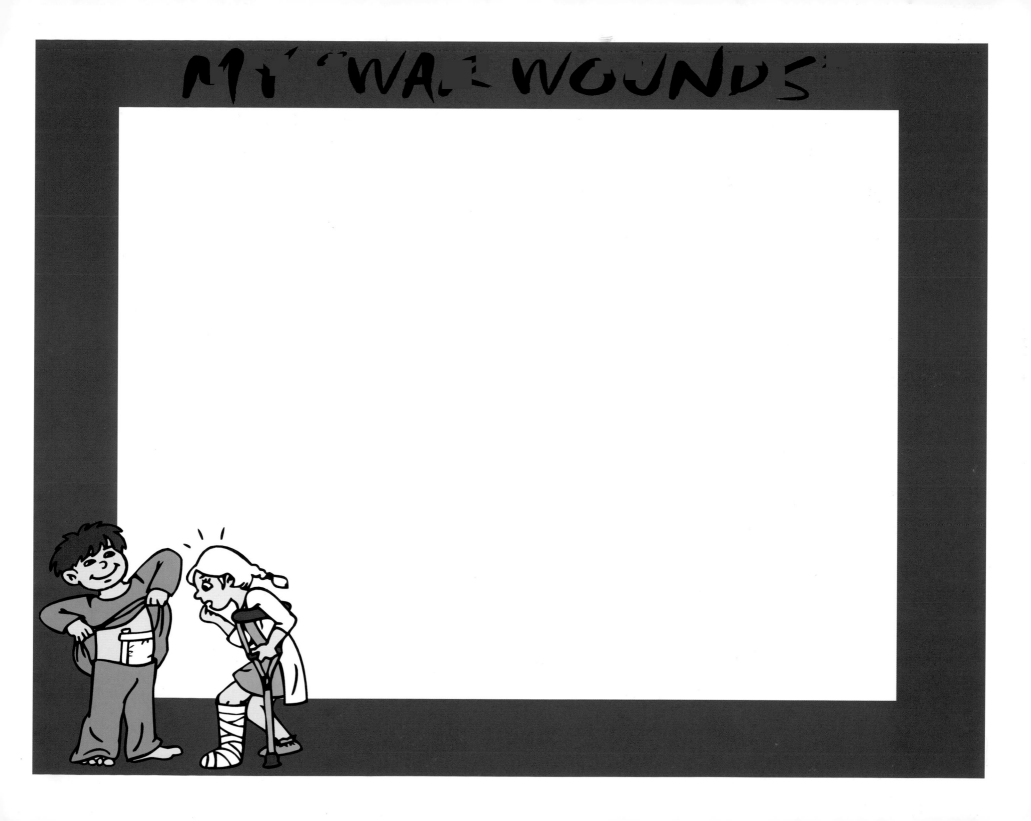

A "Good Day" Journal Entry

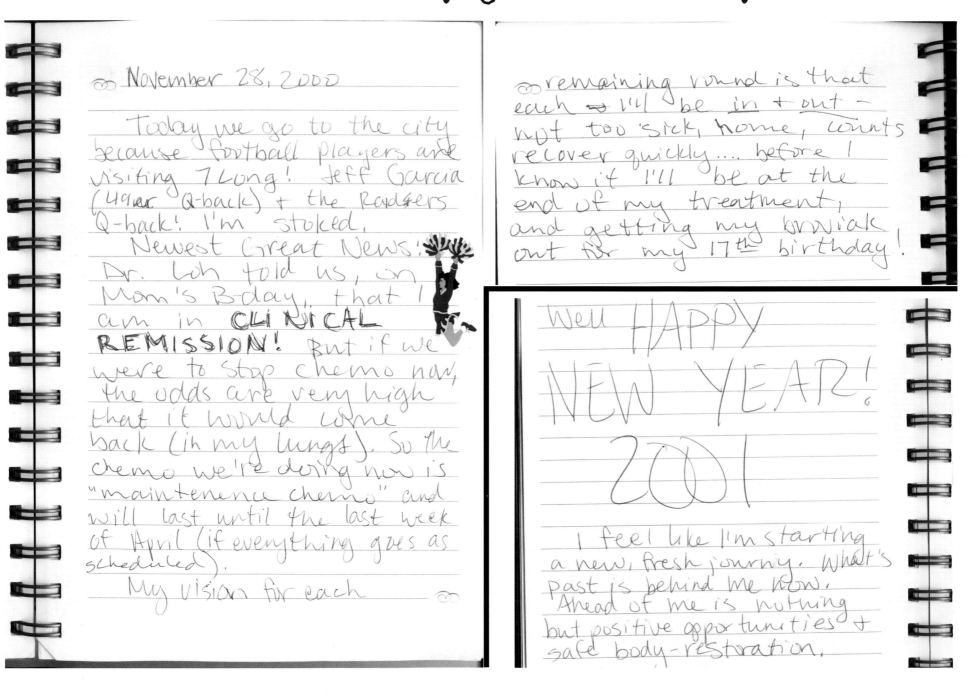

November 28, 2000

Today we go to the city because football players are visiting 7Long! Jeff Garcia (49er Q-back) + the Raiders Q-back! I'm stoked.

Newest Great News: Dr. Loh told us, on Mom's B-day, that I am in **CLINICAL REMISSION**! But if we were to stop chemo now, the odds are very high that it would come back (in my lungs). So the chemo we're doing now is "maintenance chemo" and will last until the last week of April (if everything goes as scheduled).

My vision for each

remaining round is that each → I'll be _in_ + _out_ — not too sick, home, counts recover quickly.... before I know it I'll be at the end of my treatment, and getting my broviak out for my 17th birthday!

Well **HAPPY NEW YEAR!** 2001

I feel like I'm starting a new, fresh journey. What's past is behind me now. Ahead of me is nothing but positive opportunities + safe body-restoration.

Today is a good day: _____

Today is a good day: _____

Today is a good day: _____

A "Not-So-Good Day" Journal Entry

day: Friday
date: June 9, 2000
time: 8:45am

I woke up and my esophogus was hurting so bad. I suppose it must be my esophogus, though it almost feels like it's my central line - with pressure on it or something. It's "positional" meaning it can't flow well if I'm not in a certain position - or my left side propped up w/ a pillow, so slightly on my right side, + my left arm up above my head. Oh + my left leg bent up. So that sucks.

I got a "bolis"? - morphin boost - for my pain this morning. I slept for a long time - 6am - 8:30am. Then I woke up + wanted apple

day:
date:
time:

sauce, I ate 2 bites + I started to have the same pain again. I just got another boliss, and I feel better, but it still pisses me off that it hurts to eat - even swallow my spit.

5:45 PM

I'm just kind of down today. Mom + dad are at seth's graduation - it starts at 6:30 so they're probably getting all ready to go about now. Sonia has been here, + Kathy 7-0 + Laura Dee just got here to replace Sonia. I feel bad for not having a good attitude right now. I just want to sleep - and cry but that hurts.

Today is a not-so-good day: _____

Today is a not-so-good day: _____

Today is a not-so-good day: _____

My mom made me this poster (originally 2 feet by 3 feet) as a map of everything I needed to get back to my healthy self.
It was therapeutic for her to make, as well as an interesting reminder of what I needed to get better.
...you can create your own with the next page...

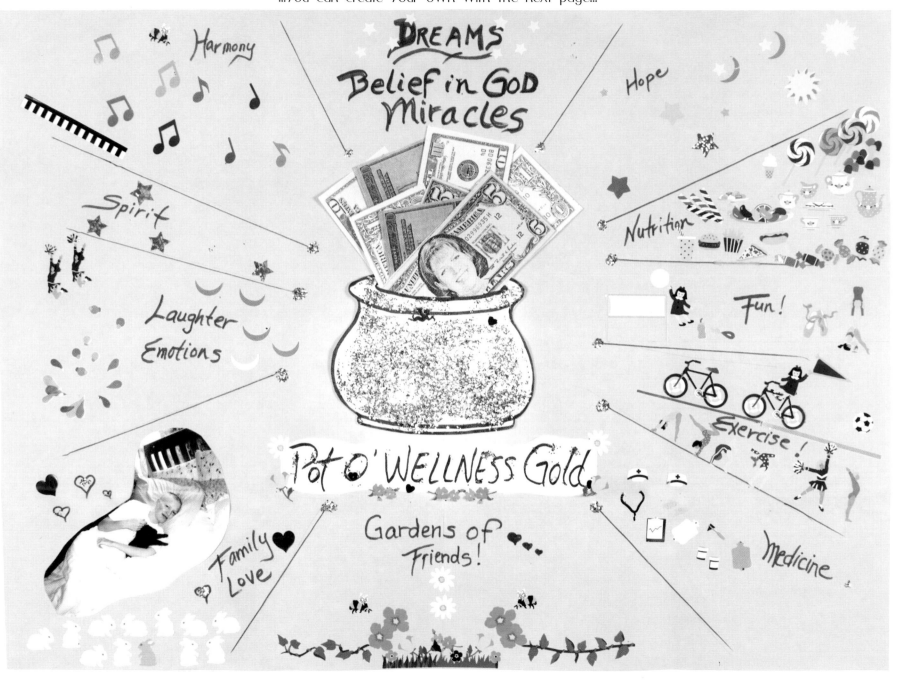

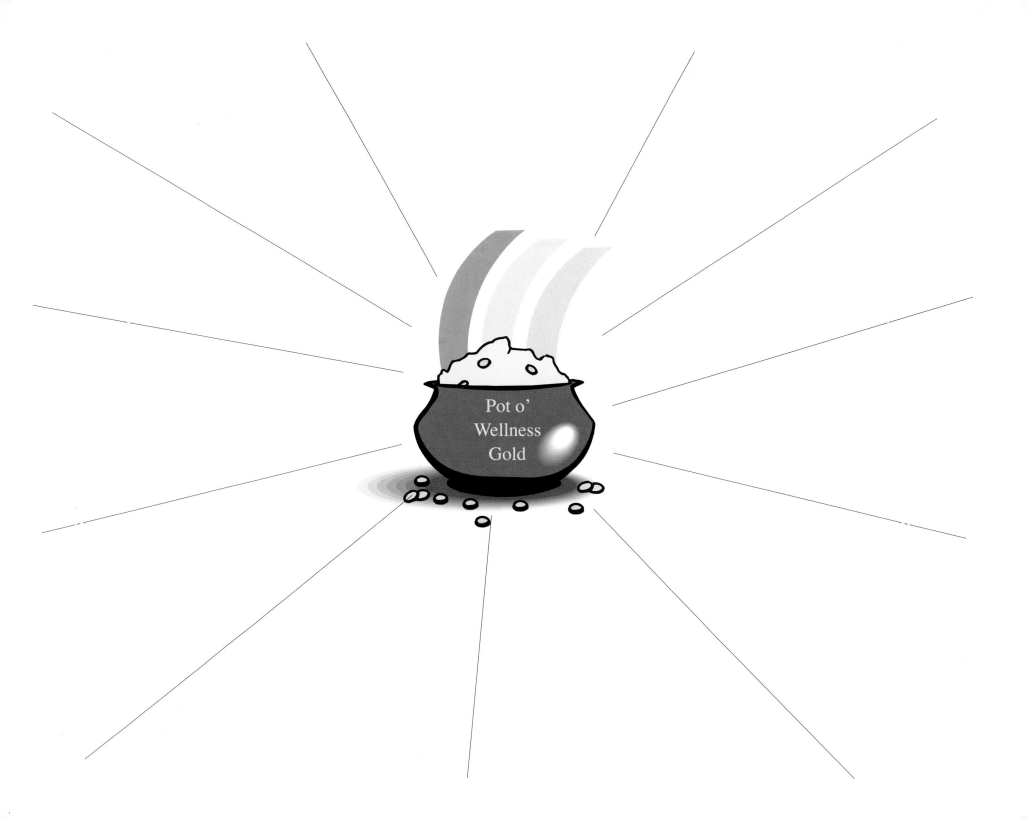

When I was on drugs, I found it extremely entertaining to color these 'trippy' pictures. They are time consuming yet fun, and provide something to do during long hours in the hospital. I also began to play around with drawing with the help of self-teaching books. Find a hobby that is fun but doesn't require too much brain power!

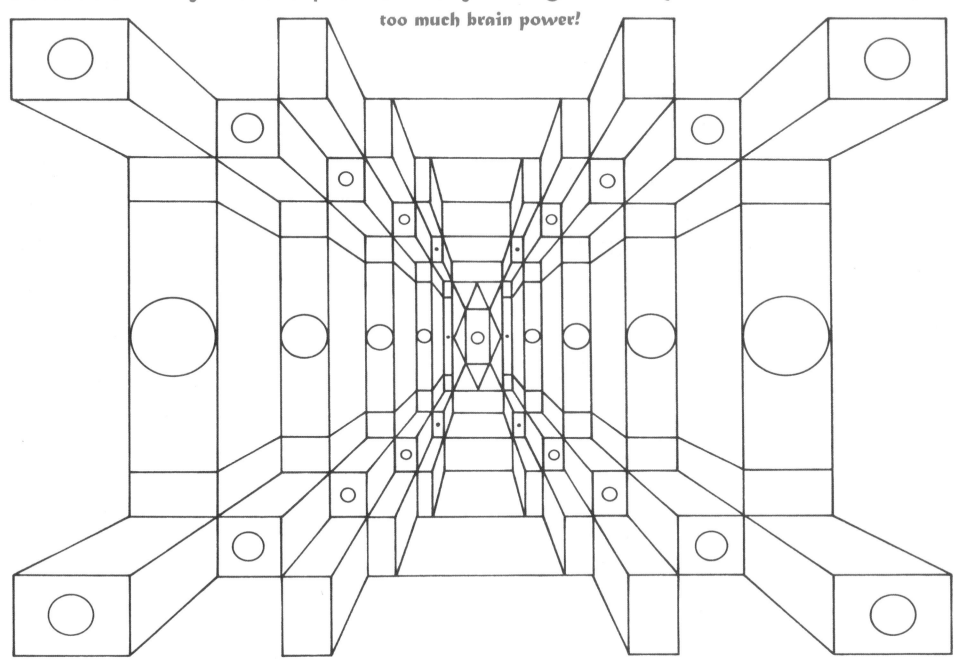

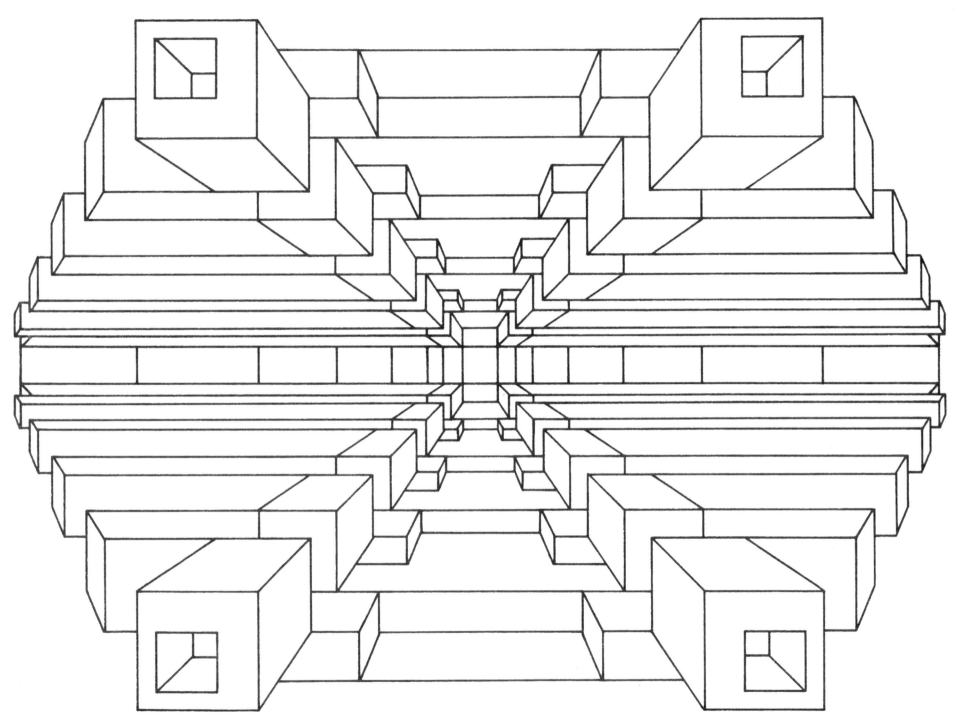

Spyros Horemis: Visual Illustions Coloring Book; Dover Publications, Inc., New York

*The following nine pages are a research paper I wrote on the benefits of determiniation and laughter (among other things) during cancer treatments. The main message is to give yourself the best quality of life possible while in treatments. This means doing everything in **your** power to improve each day, each moment.*

It is a long paper, so take your time reading it whenever you are ready!

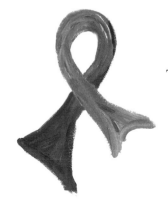

Treating Cancer with Optimism

Aubrie Maze

December 20, 2001

Senior Project Research Paper

The diagnosis of a serious disease is life shattering; it blows apart all that you know and challenges everything you have ever believed. When diagnosed with cancer, your reality is certainly shaken; on top of which exists the suffering from the affects of vigorous treatments to destroy the cancer. Being diagnosed with cancer is a fight for life, a process that social worker Beatie Lazard describes as being "put in front of Mount Everest, barefoot, at 2:00 in the morning, and being told, 'Here, climb this' " (Lazard). Cancer treatment is a most difficult, trying time for any person diagnosed, but it is amazing what you can overcome. While there are many factors that will determine your final outcome, choosing to have an upbeat attitude and a perseverance to fight your disease is crucial. Attitude will affect your state of mind, body and spirit in a positive manner, as well as improve your quality of life during your period of treatment.

The importance of conventional medicines and treatments is vital to survival. These proven methods of treatments are the choice of doctors because they are scientifically tested and confirmed to be the methods that work to combat this aggressive self-destruction of the body. The reference to conventional treatments may have a bad connotation with some people because of all the negative side affects that occur during treatments. What is now seen as the conventional, predicable, tried, and true treatments were once the radical new experiments but gained their status as the norm because they *worked.* Over the past thirty years the 'radical' approaches were sorted out to what we have now. One day a new approach to reverse the cancer cells' rapid multiplication will be discovered and solutions we do not even know will be revealed. In the meantime, the current treatments prove to be the best for our status of technology. Breast cancer survivor Lillie Shockney believes that while "biofeedback, … visual imagery… as well as an occasional therapeutic massage… helped [her] even when [she] was fighting [her cancer], [she] wouldn't be here today if [she] had shunned conventional medical care. Surgery, radiation, chemotherapy, and hormonal medication can all be absolutely crucial to a [person's] chance for long-term survival" (Shockney). The importance of oncologists and their treatments are not to be diminished: they are the cure of the majority of people diagnosed with cancer.

There are additional treatments necessary for your well-being as a whole. Lillie Shockney believes that "the exclusive use of 'alternative' remedies only creates victims. That's why [she] prefers to view those remedies as various forms of *complementary* medicine. In other words, they're treatments that pick up where medical science leaves off, but they don't conflict with it" (Shockney). This may include taking such supplements as vitamins, glyconutrients, phytonutrients or antioxidants to boost the immune system and strengthen your body to aid in its own fight, as well as such remedies as exercising your laughter, finding gratitude, and choosing optimism. These aspects are important because "in order for cancer to be a turning point, the physical, psychological, and spiritual aspects of the person must be treated in order to restore and maintain health" (Bolen, 190). All aspects of treatments can aid in your return to health. "Just about anything that fosters a positive attitude can be good medicine. The key is to include your doctor in your decisions so nothing interferes with your prescribed treatment… The best form of complementary medicine is a good attitude, especially a good sense of humor. [It is important to] inject a little humor into an otherwise grim situation because … it can make a difference in how well a patient does" (Shockney). Attitude changes your perspective on any situation, and a positive attitude can only better a circumstance.

It is reasonable for you to experience a dark side during your journey through treatments because cancer itself may be a life or death struggle, but it is dangerous when you become completely absorbed in anger, bitterness, or resentment: dwelling in such feelings can cause detriment to your health. Joanne DiNardo, a two-time cancer survivor, says that it is not beneficial to "sit in a corner and sulk or cry. That won't help you get better" (Survivor). While it is normal to have a dark side during your time in treatments and has its importance acknowledged, it is vital to balance that attitude with its opposite: a useful tool called optimism. Some think "women facing a diagnosis of breast cancer often feel pressure to maintain an optimistic attitude in order to 'beat it,' [and] this expectation may be putting an unrealistic burden on them because it's normal to feel down at times during illness and treatment" (Study). It is necessary for cancer patients to acknowledge that they may feel angry or sad at times. Drugs alone can wreak havoc on your moods, but it is also essential that you work to keep optimism and gratitude in your life.

Some cancer patients focus on their own zone of determination and drive when times become tougher. When cancer survivor Joanne DiNardo found that anger was taking her nowhere, she changed her attitude and decided she "had to be as aggressive as [her] cancer" (Survivor). DiNardo found determination, perseverance and courage. When cancer tries to destroy a person, he or she must fight back with equal or greater aggression in order to beat it. Courage is facing the challenge of a diagnosis and moving forward through treatments. "For many, [a diagnosis] mobilizes an inner warrior, and taps into a wish to live. The cancer then serves as a wake-up call to the importance of life, and in the process of coping with the cancer, the patient discovers strengths she never knew she had" (Bolen, 50-51). Cancer patients have the opportunity to realize the true value of life, and a desire to seize this newly appreciated life. The story of one cancer survivor, referred to only as "Miss Bertha," is an example of a patient with an extraordinary attitude and a courageous will to survive. When diagnosed with cancer she "was told she only had a few months to live, with an eight percent chance of survival. [She said,] '*Some* women have to make up that tiny percentage [of cancer survivors], and I intend to be one of them.' … She then went on to live another 21 years to the age of 74" (Shockney). Miss Bertha was one woman who chose not to become a victim of her cancer. Although sometimes there are no treatments to cure a cancer patient, choosing to take control of what is possible will have an enormous effect on you.

Tales told to yourself can support your mind and, thus, affect your entire body. Encouraging stories are an example of the "remarkable effect that mind can have on the body, [and] of what can happen when mind believes and matter conforms to this new belief" (Bolen, 105). Bodies operate from the messages received from the brain; when the brain believes it is doing well, the body also believes it is doing well. "The inspirational stories we hear and believe and apply to ourself get into the marrow of our bones to influence healing and recovery. The cells of the body respond, through peptide receptor sites, to true stories of remarkable recoveries, stories that are metaphors for what the body is capable of doing when we have a positive emotional response to these stories. They are transmitted in ways that we are just learning of—as energy or biochemical reactions—to activate or inspire the healing response" (Bolen, 144). When you are optimistic and tell yourself you are feeling well, your brain relays that message on to your body where your cells believe it. When a body is told that it is healthy, it responds favorably. Sometimes it may be a lie to tell your own body that you feel well, but the constant positive reinforcement still produces the same positive effects. "Affirmations are repetitive positive statements we make to ourselves… They program the current situation positively and assume success. Repetition literally changes the structure of the brain… Theoretical physicist David Bohen said, 'Any thought which is repetitious, strong, full of powerful emotion, and a sense of absolute certainty…will leave 'grooves' in the brain.'… Affirmations are a conscious effort to program the mind, often as an antidote to negative statements…or perhaps to counter one's own pessimism" (Bolen, 152-153). With sufficient effort, you may truly have the power to change yourself.

To be proactive for yourself, to take control of what you can, to be courageous, to not fall victim to your disease is vital. If you become a victim it is as if you have no control over what is happening. In reality, you *are* the one with all the choice. If you *choose* the conventional treatments, you should receive them acknowledging that you are in choice to beat your cancer. Lawrence LeShan, Ph.D., says that "it is important to remember that you are not responsible for becoming ill, and you are not responsible for your recovery. What you are responsible for once you are ill is to do your best to get better. This means getting the best medical treatment possible *and* changing your life so that your inner healing abilities will be stimulated at the highest level possible" (LeShan, xii). As a cancer patient, you must be, to a large extent, open to receive your treatments. It is not beneficial to resist medications or treatments because that would be working against them. While final outcomes cannot always be controlled, you can do your best to improve your attitude and quality of life.

Choosing to see situations in a negative light might inadvertently seem the normal route, but the angle with the positive perspective is the beneficial one. One breast cancer support group, the Johns Hopkins Breast Center, puts much effort in finding ways to fully support a cancer patient. One complementary approach they practice "involves helping each woman who undergoes [a] mastectomy to view it not as a disfiguring operation, but rather as 'transformational' surgery. The surgeon is transforming her from a victim into a survivor; she has exchanged her breast for another chance at life" (Shockney). This is an amazing and courageous way to *choose* to see a normally unfavorable situation in a positive light. Choosing the encouraging viewpoint allows for more optimism that permits you to feel better about, and generally more comfortable with, your body and yourself. If you participate in this viewpoint, you gain a new level of acceptance for yourself.

A healthy immune system helps you in your own fight for life. The challenge is that while battling cancer, you have a suppressed immune system; you must therefore have an inner change "to stimulate your immune system… There must be a change in [your] fundamental attitude toward [yourself]—toward a strong belief that you are worth fighting for and taking care of as a special, unique person with your own special ways of being, relating, and creating" (LeShan, xi-xii). LeShan also stresses that "thoughts and feelings do not cause and cannot cure cancer. But they are [an important] factor…in the total ecology that makes up a human being. Feelings affect body chemistry (which affects the development or regression of a tumor), just as body chemistry affects feelings… The immune system is strongly affected by feelings, and…taking certain kinds of psychological action can affect the immune system positively" (LeShan, xiv). There is a connection between mind, body, and soul; affirmations demonstrate this link. The power of the mind is amazing, proving that you do have some control over your situation, and you can directly contribute to your health and chance at survival.

Laughter is one of those feelings that affect your body's chemistry. To keep humor in each day and seek the fun in life will aid immensely in your fight because laughter lightens the heavy load being carried on your shoulders. The single act of laughing releases an enormous amount of bottled up emotions. The more laughter in your life, the lighter your load becomes. Humor provides contrast for the dark, depressed moments, and gives balance to an otherwise angry and bitter world. Laughter is an extreme relief that will help you as well as those around you to know that "cancer isn't a death sentence, it's a life wish" (Survivor). A diagnosis of cancer does not have to be an end of life for everyone. If you receive your diagnosis and choose to fight for your life, there will be much you will have the opportunity to learn and grow from. "Attitude is half the battle. You become what you believe and when you are laughing, you are believing in the power of life. Laughter [makes] an enormous difference to…attitude and…survival" (If). Laughing can sprout from a variety of enjoyable acts whether it be various forms of entertainment or the company of a friend. The point is to raise your level of energy and relieve your mind of the trauma it is suffering through.

Gratitude is perhaps the most valuable lesson to be received from a battle with cancer. A bout with cancer forces not only you, but also those around you, to put priorities into perspective, to see what is truly important in life. Anyone faced with a life-threatening circumstance has the opportunity to value each day more richly from the first-hand realization of how quickly and unexpectedly life can be taken away. One cancer survivor says she has "since learned to laugh often, to see [her] glass as half full rather than half empty, and to value each day" (Shockney). One faced with death realizes the value of life. Mary Cullen, a former discharge nurse at UCSF Children's Hospital who worked with cancer patients and their families every day, said that she saw "the best of people at the worst of times" (Cullen). People with cancer and those around them have a special gratitude for life once it has been threatened. In treatments, the best and worst of your character is commonly revealed. Any appalling aspects of your character allows you to appreciate the pleasant portion of yourself. After seeing this spiteful side, it is common to spend effort focusing on your pleasurable qualities. Gratitude comes in many forms, and an infinite number of items can be found each day for which to be grateful.

It is important to obtain the most possible out of life. Anyone faced with a life-threatening circumstance has the opportunity to see life in a new light. "The Chinese pictograph for *crisis* is comprised of the ideograms for 'danger' and 'opportunity' " (Bolen, 9). While your life is threatened, the opportunity arises to become a stronger, more confident, well-rounded, optimistic, and appreciative individual. "Illness is both soul-shaking and soul-evoking… You lose an innocence, you know vulnerability, you are no longer who you were before this event, and you will never be the same" (Bolen, 14). Any person who has dealt with cancer acquires something special. Survivors see what is truly important to them, and prioritize their lives differently than those who take any aspect of life for granted. In life, everyone lives with an illusion of certainty. People continue through their busy lives making plans for well in the future; but when you live with cancer, that security of certainty and planning vanishes. You lose your illusion of certainty through which the busy world operates because you can never be sure when, for example, a rush to the hospital might be necessary. Once realizing this comfort is lost, you must reintegrate planning for forward motion without quitting or giving up your life. "Life-threatening illness is a crisis for the soul… Soul questions arise about the meaning of life when the mind is ill or the body is ailing" (Bolen 9-10). Most cancer patients desire to have an insight into life. It is crucial to be determined to fight for your life, but in order to be excited about this struggle, you must know what you are fighting for.

When taken with optimism and determination, a battle with cancer can be a life-altering event, a "turning point" in life (LeShan, 180). Some may leave their battle with cancer choosing anger and bitterness, but there are those that realize the valuable lessons that can be taken from such an experience. Those that survive their cancer and recognize the value to be found continue on to live a meaningful life: enjoying their life and helping others find the same joy. Because as a cancer patient, you are forced to the edge of life, you have the opportunity to discover your purpose in life. It is after such an experience that most people are inspired to grasp that opportunity to live their life's purpose.

Cancer strikes all aspects of a human being. It doesn't miss any side of being human. It affects mind, body, and spirit. It shakes you to the core. Once surviving this attack, you will be strengthened because each part of you fought and won. "People who survive a life-threatening illness, which becomes a turning point in their lives, have come through a transformative soul experience as well as a physical crisis" (Bolen 180). In order to maintain life, you must reach down into the depth of your being to find grit and courage to wage the battle.

> A life-threatening illness brings suffering and soul into our lives. It brings us close to the bone as it strips us of nonessentials and insignificant concerns. It makes us aware of how short life is and how precious good moments are, and connects us to others and to the suffering that only compassionate acts can alleviate. If it does not kill us, it indeed makes us strong. Times of crisis are opportunities for accelerated lessons in what it is to be human. Assuming that we are spiritual beings on a human path, rather than human beings on a spiritual path, then the most difficult times in our lives also teach us and test us and often pull us back onto a soul track or a heart path—often, when we thought we were lost. It is a time when we may discover or remember once again that this human journey is much easier when we love one another, see the divinity in each other, and know we are not alone… [Bolen has] often ended a lecture or workshop by playing a simple song…by John Denver, because his words tell it all—they tell us about the ingredients of life and the fullness of it. I suggest you read it slowly, out loud to yourself.
> > *All this joy, all this sorrow, all this promise, all this pain.*
> > *Such is life, such is being, such is spirit, such is love.*   (Bolen, 210).

Though no one would wish cancer on another, the gifts from the journey can be amazing, and can only be gained from such a trial. The gifts from a battle with cancer can be as profound as the journey itself. What is done "between being born and dying is what matters. The point…is to live a meaningful life, however long or short it may be. If a life-threatening illness or a chronic disabling illness is what the soul encounters, then this is the current shape of the soul journey" (Bolen, 204). Seeking solutions through the wisdom of those who have previously encountered similar obstacles is an avenue of valuable resource through which to persevere and maintain an optimistic attitude. Choosing laughter and optimism, courage and determination, will aid in your battle. Looking for the gifts, regardless of the packaging, allows you to be propelled through each day, moment by moment.

Works Cited

Bolen, Jean Shinoda (M.D.). <u>Close to the Bone: Life-Threatening Illness and the Search for Meaning</u>. New York: Touchstone, 1996.

Cullen, Mary (Former discharge nurse at UCSF Medical Center). Personal interview. 9 December 2001.

"If There's A Key to Survival, It's Laughter, Survivor Says." [Online]. Available <u>www.cancer.org</u>. Retrieved 14 October 2001

Lazard, Beatrix (Beatie) (Social Worker at UCSF Medical Center). Telephone interview. 6 December 2001.

LeShan, Lawrence (Ph.D,). <u>Cancer As A Turning Point: A Hand book for People with Cancer, Their Families, and Health Professionals: Revised Edition</u>. New York: Plume, 1994

Shockney, Lillie (RN, BS, MAS). "Breast Cancer: Alternative Medicine and an Upbeat Attitude." [Online]. Available <u>www.mothersdaughters.org/medicine.html</u>. Retrieved14 October 2001.

"Study Examines Emotions and Breast Cancer Survival." [Online]. Available <u>www.cancer.org</u>. Retrieved 14 October 2001.

"Survivor Learns to Sprinkle Bad News With Laughter." [Online]. Available <u>www.cancer.org</u>. Retrieved 14 October 2001.

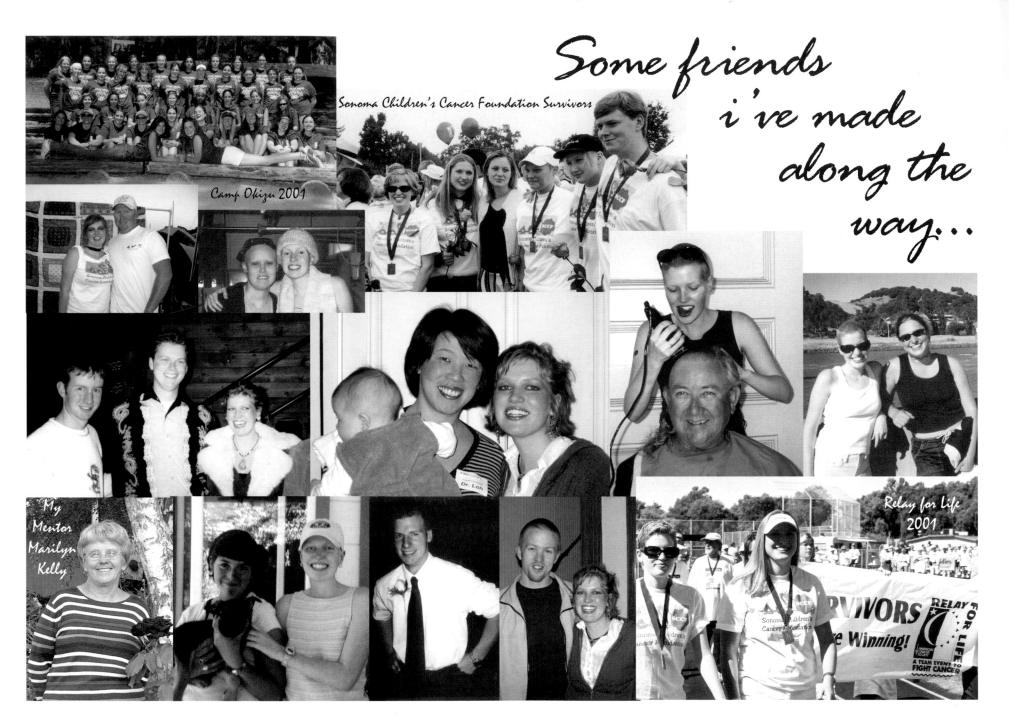

Some friends
i've made
along the
way...

Sonoma Children's Cancer Foundation Survivors

Camp Okizu 2001

My
Mentor
Marilyn
Kelly

Relay for Life
2001

Although the journey was a difficult one, the friends I've made along the way are priceless.
Having cancer opens up a whole new world; one I will never shy away from.

Friends I Have Made During My Journey:

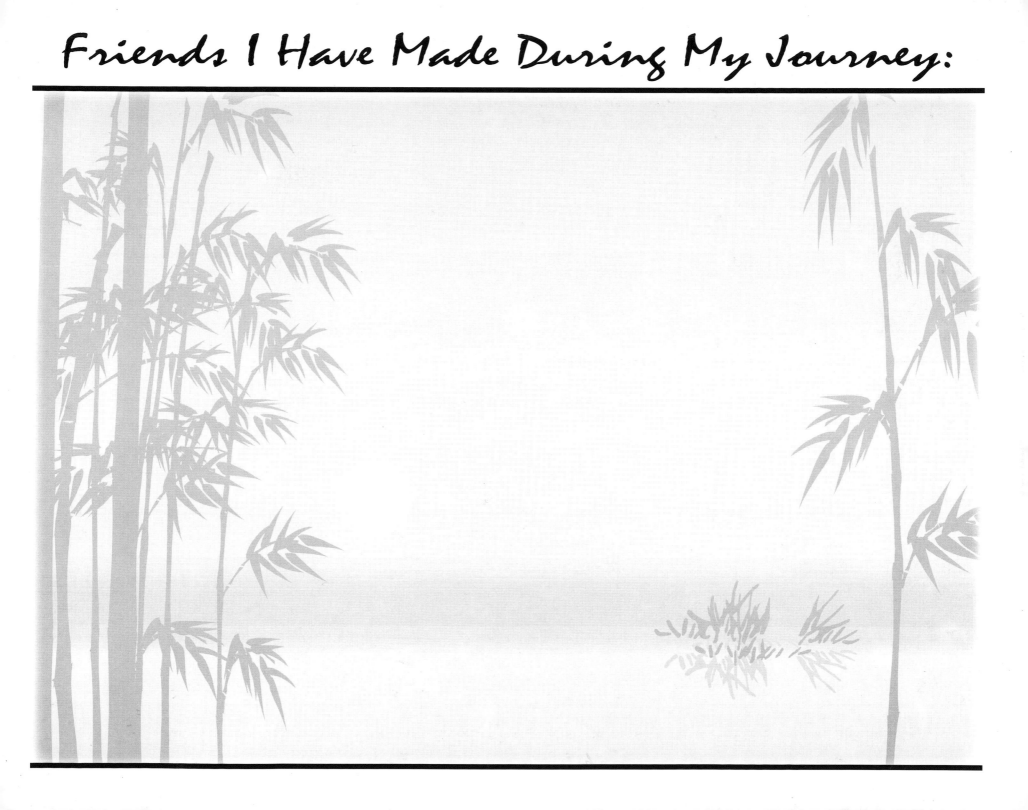

"Courage Is The Thing With Claws"

Courage is the thing with claws

That lives deep inside you.

It rips its way out when it smells fear

And forces your soul through.

Although it takes every piece of you

To go that extra mile.

Your courage will really shine through

When you still have time to smile.

I love you Aubrie!

With Love,

Meghan Sullivan

"Work like you don't need the money.

Love like you've never been hurt.

Dance like no one is watching."

- Author Unknown

Your battle with cancer is unique to you.

Give it your all.

Deepest Blessings,

Aubrie Maze

epilogue

(ONE YEAR POST DIAGNOSIS)
Email to Friends and Family:
June 1st, 2001

Happy Friday –

I'm not sure if my mom wrote to tell you about our conversations the other day with my oncologist, Dr. Loh. Dr. Loh said she thought maybe I was done with chemo since my platelets just were not coming up – like maybe my body is trying to tell me something... (Which was very ironic because my mom, her sister, and a good friend of ours all had the same thought.) That definitely scared me... but I was also disappointed because I wanted the whole celebrations around GOING IN FOR MY LAST TREATMENT, and all that. So she said we'd do one more round, and "call it a day," meaning be done with it.

We did a blood draw this morning, for a possible Saturday afternoon admission. (Afternoon because my SAT's are in the morning!) Well, Dr. Loh just called me and told me that my platelets are still at 74,000, (and they need to be at 100,000 for chemo). So no potatoes – (no go). We'll do another blood draw Tuesday, and see how my counts are. If my platelets are high enough, then we'll go in for one last round of chemo. But if they haven't come up enough, then that will be the end of my treatments, and I'll be in REMISSION.

It seems I've waited so long for this time, but I'm not excited. I'm scared. Maybe I'm scared because we're finishing early, and I'm scared it's not enough. But it obviously is enough if my bone marrow is too tired to make more platelets. Dr. Loh said she needs to make sure I get adequate treatments, but she also needs to look out for my long term health – and more chemo when I might not be able to recover is not good. And the point of chemo is to be given a lot, frequently, to surprise any cancer cells. If you wait 4 or 5 or 6 weeks between chemo, it does nothing but poison your body. I suppose I'm also scared because this lifestyle has become normal and safe for me. Going back into what everyone else's normal world is a scary thing. I don't know. I'm not sure what I'm feeling. I'll let you know when I figure it out.

I'll write soon. Thank you for your continued prayers.

Love,

Aubrie

Email to Friends and Family:
June 5th, 2001

Hi!!

I just wanted to jot a quick note to tell you some exciting news we received today from my oncologist, Dr. Loh. And that is... I AM DONE WITH ALL OF MY TREATMENTS!!! Full REMISSION. Wow. Just wow. Now we're ready to celebrate. It's funny that a huge lesson this past year has been how unreliable "planning" is. We always try to plan out the future – even just the day. But this last year, we have had to totally learn to not count on any of our plans. Just about the time we'd think "Oh, well we know for sure this week is free...", I'd come down with a fever or something and have to be rushed to the hospital for a week's stay. So again, we actually thought we could plan something – we thought we could plan when I'd be done. (We knew for SURE I'd go in sometime...) And then my body turns around and says "No... I think I've had enough." So we're ending this journey on the same unexpected and unpredictable note as we started. You'd think we would have learned our lesson by now, but no... :)

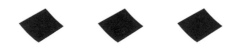

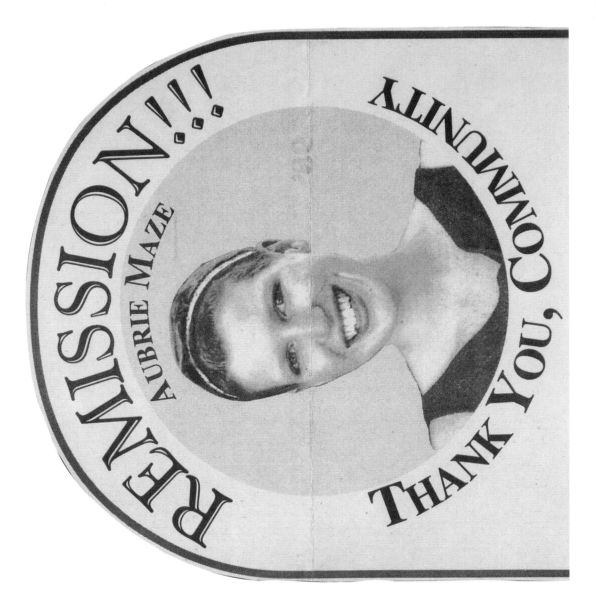

REMISSION!!!

AUBRIE MAZE

THANK YOU, COMMUNITY

Some thank you's for the production of this book:

to Mom: for your support in the early morning, late night, and all the hours in between, and for your never ending determination to keep this project manage to show up at the perfect time and place, with the perfect advice; to John Delaplaine: for your ability to keep me continuously inspired with for your guidance as my Senior Project mentor; to Lilla and Andy Weinberger (aka, Readers' Books): for hosting my very first book talk and signing!; to the (who wish to remain anonymous): the physical production of this book would not have been possible without you; to everyone who gave me feedback and new shape or form: thank you, thank you, thank you. You have all been gusts of wind

To all of you who held her in your hearts for all this time, we thank you.

To those of you who prayed for her and held the vision for her healing, we thank you.

To God, and our relationship with Him:

through whom all our inspiration and strength comes, we thank You.

Thank ALL of you who: created and organized fundraisers of an amazing variety for her, worked their tails off for them and to those who came to them and gave so graciously. Those who donated your places for events for her, who ran and walked marathons in her name, wrote articles about her and published them. Who danced for her, sang for her, did magic shows for her, sold programs for her and those who stepped up to lead the effort. Those who did car washes and shared your fundraisers with her, wrote emails and letters to keep our families and friends updated when we could not, who gave money for our family, managed the donations and wrote the 'thank yous'. Bought presents for her, wrote cards and letters for her, made drawings, wrote songs and poems for her. And to those who wrote and drew for her daily. Those who gave her hats and scarves, and those who made them for her. Those who cooked and baked for her, treated us to your restaurants when she could be out, brought her food at home and in the hospital. Who read to her, sang to her, sat with her and talked with her-or not. Told stories to her, encouraged her, watched movies with her, and ate with her when she could. To those wonders who threw a graduation party for her brother 3 weeks after she was diagnosed and to those who made her feel safe while we were gone. Who tutored her in her classes, provided extras to make school work more do-able, fought for her, bought and sold raffle tickets for her, and to those who made it possible for her to win THAT car! Those who paid our bills, opened up their homes, did energy body work on her, massaged her- but not too hard - and held her. To you who asked her to throw the first pitch out at her high school baseball game when she was ready-to include her. To those who did the lab work for her, tests for her, organized and delivered medical supplies to her. To those who raised awareness of her, called her, emailed her, created a website for her and to those who manage it. Who sent your email about her on to others to widen the prayer circle for her and to those who made that circle go around the world. To those who made her feel good about herself, made her laugh, made her forget for even just one minute what she was going through. To those who cared for her in her darkest times -all you angels at Sonoma Valley Hospital and USCF & the 7 Long Oncology Team. We will never forget you.

To those who never gave up hope for her. To those of you who are still asking about her.

To all of you, impossible to list, we thank you.

Aubrie is complete with all her treatments, looks and feels fabulous and is ready to take on the world!!

This has been so Powerful.

You have touched our Hearts and Souls forever.

Thank you

Rick, Kristin, Seth & Aubrie Maze

www.aubriespage.com

---

rolling; to Daddy and Seth: for being my constant backbone of support; to all my family: for being my foundation; to Julia Challonar: you always

your savvy computer problem solving; to Carol Salvin: you brought my book to a whole new level and made my dream a reality; to Marilyn Kelly:

Sonoma Children's Cancer Foundation: you have kept me intimate with my experience through cancer treatments; to my generous financial contributors

ideas: you helped me see my book through new eyes; to all my angels, tall and short alike, to everyone impossible to name, who helped in any color,

in my sail. I am truly appreciative and deeply grateful to all of you.

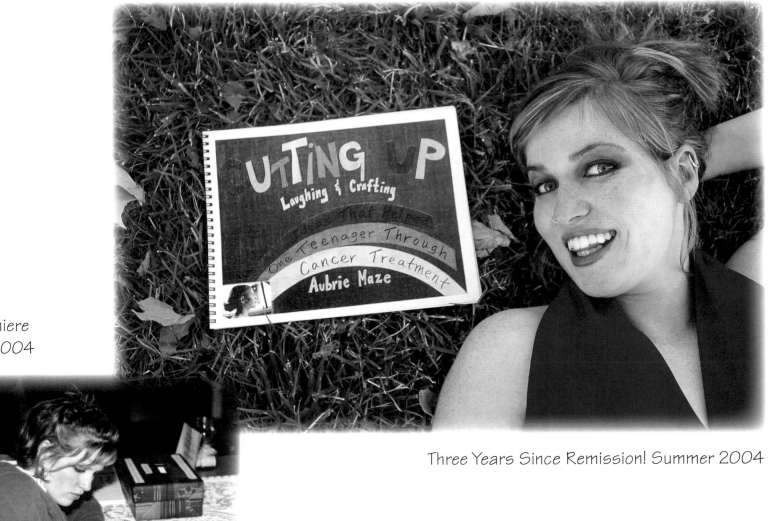

Book Premiere
January 2004

Three Years Since Remission! Summer 2004

SINCE REMISSION...

After my year in cancer treatments (including chemo, radiation, surgery...) and finally Remission (!), I made it through the hospital withdrawals I was having... into a summer filled with making up my Junior year, which I had missed while I was in treatments (except for three classes in which I was home-tutored during the end of my treatments, when I felt relatively better.) I worked my little buns off, finishing my Junior year classes just in time to start my Senior year in High School. I took on a fairly difficult load, including a 7am Pre-Calculus class, and two AP (college level) classes. Between my schoolwork (including creating this book), leadership activities and social life, I left very little time to rest and recuperate from my year in cancer treatments. Add on the pressure of applying for college and scholarships, and generally preparing myself to leave home, I completely wore myself out.

I had an amazing healing session with a Shiatsu Master, David Kukkula. He encouraged me to listen to my body; I realized I was tired and I needed a break. I also realized the only thing pushing me straight off to college were my pre-cancer-self goals, which by no means had included battling cancer.

I had a good cry, took some deep breaths, and let my shoulders drop a good two inches. For the first time in a long while, I was relaxed, not stressed, armed with a clean slate and an open mind.

I decided to take a year off school after graduating from high school. My plans were vague and I occasionally felt judged by others ("Well what are you going to **DO**?" My response: "Well... rest.") I enjoyed the rest of my Senior year; I took a two week trip to Europe; I spent some time visiting relatives; I worked fun part-time jobs; I worked on this book; I relaxed; I hung out with friends; I went to hospital checkups and scans; I celebrated anniversaries: two years since my last chemo, two years since remission, three years since diagnosis, etcetera; I recuperated from my battle with cancer: one year spent fighting, one year spent resting: seems like a fair trade, you know?

I am currently in college. I am trusting myself and my current needs and wants, not blindly following my past goals. I had always wanted to move away to college; the last place I wanted to go was the Junior College 30 minutes from my home... I am currently attending the Santa Rosa Junior College, 30 minutes from my home. The truth is, I was not ready to move away. (My plans to move to San Francisco are beginning to roll...) I am continuing to recover from a scary battle that still makes me bawl. I am doing what it takes to keep myself healthy, not stressed. I am enjoying a fun, relaxing time at school, taking classes that interest me. For the most part, my best friends are still nearby - a nice incentive to stick around. It is all enjoyable. I am finding that the recovery process is just as vital as the actual fight because it secures long term health. So take all the time you need to recover, because really, you have all the time in the world.

Slow down, take a break, really listen to yourself. Do what your heart tells you. Do what makes you happy. Enjoy life.

Good Luck and Congratulations!

Fellow Survivor,

Aubrie Maze